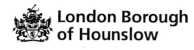

**WILFRED R. PIGEON** Ph.D.

CONSULTANT **MICHAEL J. SATEIA** MD

# *sleep*manual

how to achieve the perfect night's sleep

First published in 2010 by
New Holland Publishers (UK) Ltd
London • Cape Town • Sydney • Auckland

Garfield House
86–88 Edgware Road
London W2 2EA
United Kingdom
www.newhollandpublishers.com

80 McKenzie Street
Cape Town 8001
South Africa

Unit 1, 66 Gibbes Street
Chatswood, NSW 2067
Australia

218 Lake Road
Northcote, Auckland
New Zealand.

10 9 8 7 6 5 4 3 2 1

ISBN-13: 978-1-84773-723-6

**Important Note:** The information given in
this book is not intended as medical advice,
but rather as a tool for general guidance in
dealing with a sleep disorder. You should
always consult your doctor or other qualified
medical professional before embarking on
any treatment programme. In particular,
please note that drugs mentioned in this
book may vary from country to country, so
always check the suitability of all medications
with your doctor first. While every care has
been taken to ensure the accuracy of the
information contained in this book, neither
the publisher nor the contributors can accept
liability for any errors or omissions,
howsoever caused.

This book was conceived,
designed and produced by
**Ivy Press**
210 High Street,
Lewes,
East Sussex, BN7 2NS, UK

*Creative Director* Peter Bridgewater
*Publisher* Jason Hook
*Art Director* Michael Whitehead
*Editorial Director* Caroline Earle
*Senior Editor* Lorraine Turner
*Consultant Reader* Stephen Lund, MD
*Design* JC Lanaway

# CONTENTS

# FOREWORD

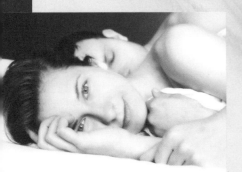

Difficulty in sleeping has plagued human beings for millennia. References to insomnia can be traced from the earliest civilizations to the Bible, down through the ages in literature and, to some extent, science. The problems related to insomnia range from mild inconvenience to life-altering, all-consuming disturbances that may fundamentally change the course of a person's existence.

Until relatively recently, medical science largely ignored sleep-related conditions such as insomnia. However, during the latter half of the twentieth century and into the twenty-first, our understanding of the nature and consequences of disordered sleep has grown exponentially. It has become clear that good-quality sleep in adequate amounts is an essential component of balanced health. Not only does poor or inadequate sleep result in the most apparent consequences of fatigue, impaired cognitive function, and reduced quality of life, but – as emerging data suggest – it may predispose to other psychological and physiological disturbances, including depression and disturbance in the cardiovascular, immune, and other biological systems.

In light of this information, increasing emphasis has been placed on the identification and treatment of chronic insomnia. Despite this, most individuals with this condition remain undiagnosed and untreated. We have come to understand that insomnia, like other disturbances of fundamental biological functions, has a specific set of causes for which there are effective therapies. Regrettably, many health-care providers receive limited education in this area, resulting in deficits of knowledge and understanding of the condition. This book – while not intended to be a substitute for adequate medical assessment and therapy – will enable those who suffer from insomnia to perceive with greater clarity the nature of their condition, to distinguish disorders and factors that contribute to their insomnia, and to identify (and, in some cases, implement) treatment. The information presented here should also serve to facilitate interaction between the health-care provider and a well-informed patient.

As you digest the information herein, it will become apparent that chronic insomnia is often a complex and multifaceted problem. So the therapeutic approach will, of necessity, be multi-dimensional in its approach. That said, Dr Pigeon has succeeded in presenting a highly accessible and thorough account of the causes and solutions for chronic insomnia, which will provide readers with considerable understanding of why their sleep is disturbed.

Building on an overview of the basic structure and characteristics of sleep, this book moves from a systematic discussion of the most common sleep disorders to a more detailed analysis of the problems that can precipitate (as well as perpetuate) chronic insomnia. In the therapy section, Dr Pigeon carefully walks the reader through a detailed 'self-assessment' of adaptive and maladaptive sleep habits that will facilitate identification and correction of many of the cognitive and behavioural factors that perpetuate sleep disturbance, long after the initial causes of insomnia have been resolved. A detailed and well-balanced overview of the array of specific pharmacological, psychological, behavioural and alternative therapies for insomnia succinctly elaborates which treatments work, which do not, and why. In the course of this discussion, several things will become clear to the reader: it is important to understand the underlying causes and contributing factors, which are unique for every person with insomnia; effective therapies are available, but must be employed in a thoughtful and specific fashion; motivation and consistency are critical in overcoming sleep disturbance.

Dr Pigeon is a highly regarded expert in the field of insomnia, especially in the application of non-pharmacological therapies. In this book he has provided people suffering from insomnia with a straightforward description of the nature of this condition, its consequences and causes. More importantly, *Sleep Manual* offers a concise and practical set of guidelines that will enable insomnia sufferers to address their sleep problems in effective ways. The message is clear: insomnia is a significant health problem. But it can be treated effectively – and now is the time to get started.

MICHAEL J. SATEIA, MD

# INTRODUCTION

Welcome to this manual and what I hope will be a transformative experience not only for your sleep life but also for your entire life. It is no secret that sleep is vital for optimal functioning and well-being. The information in this manual is also no secret, although it is seldom available in its entirety.

This manual provides the insomnia sufferer with a thorough handbook for identifying and rectifying the sleep disturbances that affect them. The first section of the book is devoted to giving you a grounding in the science of sleep, explaining the host of sleep disorders that exist, and understanding the types and consequences of insomnia. The second section is devoted to the 'how to' of developing and implementing a personalized programme to improve your sleep. The accompanying CD provides a variety of tools to help characterize the nature of your sleep problem and to structure a sleep programme tailored to your individual needs.

## WHY LEARN ABOUT SLEEP BEFORE COMMENCING THE PROGRAMME?

As you make your way through the first few chapters in this manual, you will be learning the same lessons that a sleep specialist would impart to you in the early stages of individual therapy for insomnia just as if you were sitting across from him or her in an office – lessons that insomnia experts believe set the stage for a successful course of therapy, if properly understood and applied. By knowing how the mind and body construct good sleep, you can better understand when those parts are not functioning properly. This knowledge enables you to evaluate the usefulness of the variety of treatment options available for insomnia.

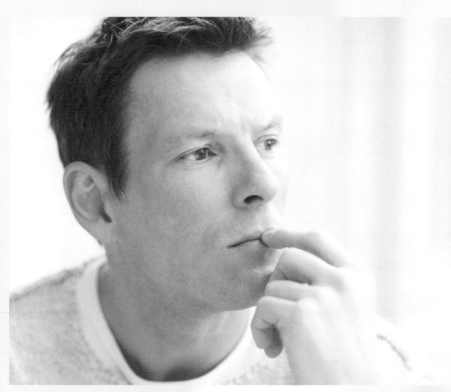

It may be tempting to skip to the second section of the manual in order to get to work, but learning about the basics of sleep is well worth the reading time. In a clinical setting, a diagnosis of insomnia is made only after the possible presence of other sleep disorders has been evaluated. Some of these disorders are so common that if you do not have one yourself, someone you know undoubtedly will. The information on the disorders in Chapter 2 may not directly apply to your current situation, but may well serve other people you know or be useful to you at a later time. Chapters 3 and 4 provide a detailed examination of insomnia and how its development and persistence can be related to the science of sleep as set out in Chapter 1, as well as how insomnia can affect various areas of your life.

ABOVE *Identifying the sleep disturbances that affect you or someone you know, and understanding their nature and causes will help you pave the way to rectifying them.*

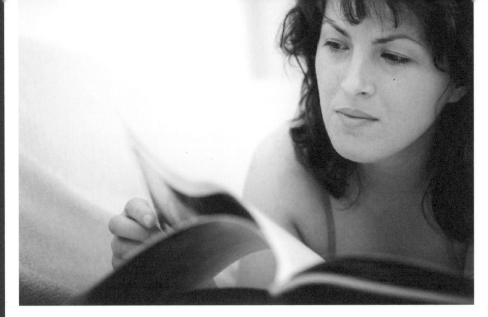

## DESIGNING A PERSONALIZED SLEEP-IMPROVEMENT PROGRAMME

The knowledge you gain from the first section of the manual will provide a foundation for building a unique sleep programme. Insomnia does not come in just one form; neither, then, should the treatment for insomnia. The main approaches suggested in this book have been empirically validated many times over. Surely a number of readers will have previously attempted to use some of these strategies, based on a magazine article or news story. There is no substitute, however, for getting the full package that this manual provides and for applying it consistently over time.

## A JOINT VENTURE

The approach in this manual relies heavily on you providing a very detailed appraisal of your sleep. In essence, you will be giving yourself an incredibly thorough sleep evaluation, guided by the manual. With this approach you become an active agent in your own care, using the resources of the manual as your partner. I have found that the patients who are most successful in addressing their insomnia are those who are actively engaged in their treatment. They ask questions and challenge the reasons for engaging in particular treatment strategies. They provide

*ABOVE  Being well informed will empower you to adopt the right approach to building a personalized sleep programme.*

feedback on how these strategies are working, bring up problems as they occur, and join with me to solve those problems. Since you have taken the initiative to begin reading this manual, you are already engaged in just such a joint venture.

## NOT ONE APPROACH, BUT MANY

The best way to address insomnia is through cognitive-behavioural therapy. However, this therapy is composed of several individual therapies. Each of these in turn can and should be modified to fit your particular circumstances. The manual provides the means for fine-tuning each piece to address specific facets of your sleep experience. In addition, Chapter 6 provides an explanation of a myriad of other treatment options that are available for insomnia, with guidelines on their possible inclusion in your programme. This includes a review of natural remedies, alternative therapies and the many sleep medications and sleep aids that are used for insomnia.

## SOME SIZES *DO* FIT ALL

In Chapter 5 you will find some strategies that are recommended regardless of your situation or insomnia type. Drawing from the groundwork laid in previous chapters, you can begin to apply these forms of therapy with renewed confidence in your ability to positively modify your sleep. Even within these general strategies there is room (and need) to tailor the approaches to the information gleaned from evaluating your sleep.

## A CUSTOM FIT

The creation of your individualized sleep programme begins in earnest with the Sleep Workshop in Chapter 7. Here you are introduced to the most powerful techniques for combating insomnia. In Chapter 8 you continue the extensive work you have done so far and rebuild, piece by piece, the structure needed for consistent good sleep. It is no small task – insomnia is no small problem, and there is no one answer. There is, however, a programme that can be tailored to your personal situation to ensure your success.

BELOW *In this book you will find detailed explanations of the treatment options that are available for insomnia and other sleep disturbances.*

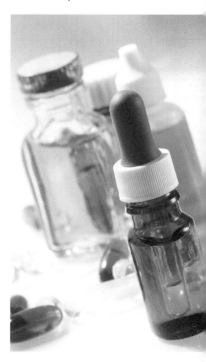

## USING THE ACCOMPANYING CD

There is a lot of work involved in constructing a truly tailored approach to treating insomnia. The tools used by insomnia experts need to be available to the people who are willing to go to the necessary lengths to design and implement their own programmes. Simply reading this book and following the instructions are not enough. Some of the tools of the trade are available within these pages, but there isn't sufficient room to include them all. Moreover, some of the tools are far more useful in their entirety than in a condensed version made to fit on the page. Other tools are useful only if they can be modified by the user. Still others are best when you interact with them in a spreadsheet format. For these reasons, the accompanying CD provides a rich set of resources to guide the creation and delivery of your sleep programme.

### CONTENT OF THE CD

The CD contains copies of all the tools provided in this book, as well as a number of additional tools, including questionnaires and checklists to help you evaluate your sleep. There are also forms to enable you to identify all the sleep factors that you

BELOW *The CD that accompanies this book contains useful tools to help you devise your own sleep programme.*

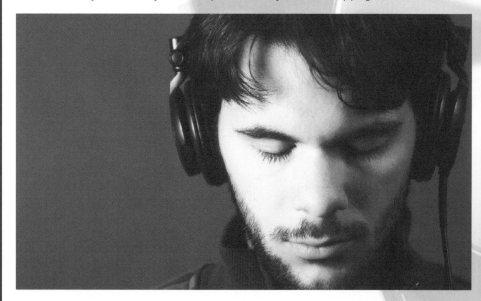

need to address regarding your particular sleep problem, and forms to help you weigh up the relative merits of including various strategies for each of these problems. Two guided relaxation exercises are also available, should you choose to use them as a piece of your treatment programme. They will help you to relax and set the right mood earlier in the day for a good night's sleep later. A calculator is also available to help you calculate important sleep variables (and an Excel version if you prefer to use Excel spreadsheets), along with graphs to track your progress as you proceed through your programme. In addition, the documents can be easily printed out from the CD so that you can write on them and keep them handy.

## HOW TO USE THE CD

The CD is best used in conjunction with the manual. Regardless of how you end up constructing your programme, I strongly recommend that you use the tools on the CD to review and track your progress. As a starting point, listen to the introduction and proceed from there.

## SOME PROMISES

Reading this manual from cover to cover will give you a deeper understanding of how sleep should work. If you also complete the questionnaires, checklists, forms and logs in the book and on the CD, you will have a clearer picture of your insomnia than when you began. You will arrive at a well-suited outcome.

There is no guarantee of treatment success, but my experience is that how you approach treatment can greatly affect the outcome. Your chances of successfully resolving your insomnia will improve dramatically if you follow and continually assess the programme that you create from this book in a rigorously consistent manner for several weeks.

**Reminder: printable versions of all forms included in this book are available on the enclosed CD.**

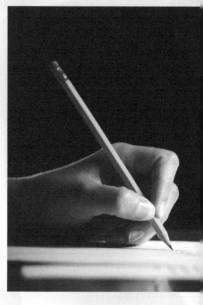

ABOVE *Making notes as you go along will help you analyse and understand your own sleep pattern and monitor your progress.*

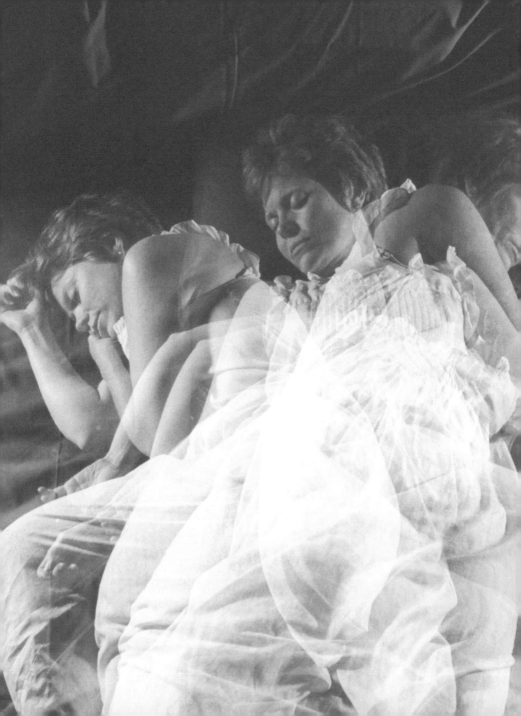

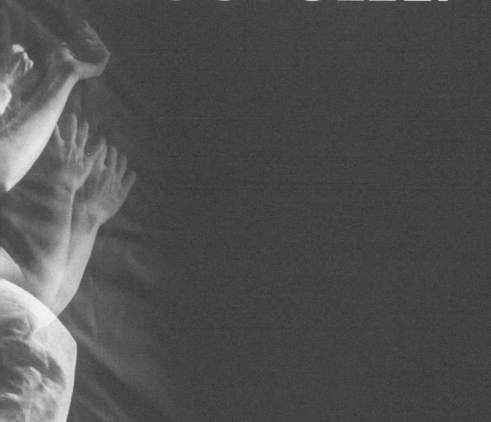

# SECTION 1
# LEARNING ABOUT SLEEP

The relatively new science of sleep has uncovered many of the intricate pieces that comprise the sleep system. In this chapter we will review what sleep is and what function it serves as well as what happens to our bodies and minds while we sleep. What is dreaming? What amount of sleep is best? Do sleep needs change over our lifetimes? The science of sleep has addressed these types of questions, and we will explore the answers.

# CHAPTER 1
# THE SCIENCE OF SLEEP

## WHAT IS SLEEP?

What is sleep? It is such a simple question. Yet this question has challenged a variety of great thinkers throughout the years and produced a multitude of perspectives. Is sleep the 'chief nourisher' in life, as the playwright William Shakespeare wrote, or is it 'perverse as human nature', as depicted by the poet Ogden Nash? The answer, as in so much of life, is both. Today, you would think that modern science would be more precise. Yet pose this question to three sleep researchers and you will elicit a set of related yet totally unique responses. Let us explore, however, what these researchers are most likely to agree on.

BELOW *Experts' opinions vary, but most now agree that sleep is not a suspension of consciousness but an active conscious state.*

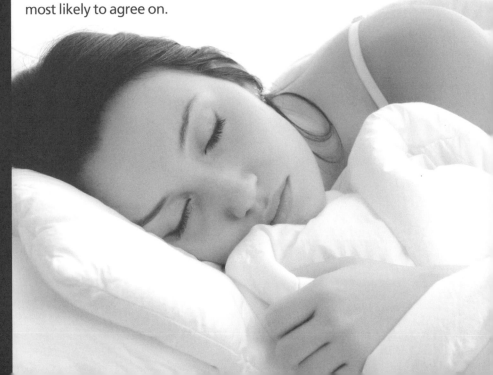

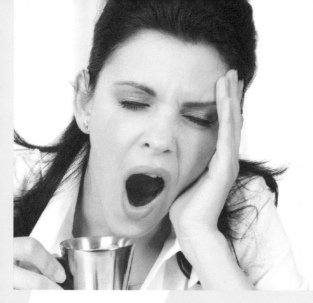

LEFT *Most people agree that a lack of nourishing sleep leads to fatigue and drowsiness during the daytime.*

## SLEEP AS AN ABSENCE OF WAKEFULNESS

In the twentieth century it was widely believed that sleep was a progressive withdrawal from wakefulness and the waking world. Merriam-Webster's dictionary described it as 'a periodic suspension of consciousness', a state of hibernation, if you will, somewhere between waking and death, in which not a whole lot was happening. This fitted the available evidence that basic physiological processes slow down as we enter sleep. The heart rate decreases, breathing slows down and brain waves, which were first measured in humans in Germany in 1927, also slow down when we close our eyes. The notion that sleep was simply being 'unawake' also fitted in with most personal experiences of sleep as a cessation of mental activity.

## SLEEP AS AN ACTIVE CONSCIOUS STATE

In 1936, the first electroencephalographic (EEG) recording of sleep in humans took place at Harvard Medical School. What was observed led to a major paradigm shift. The sleeping EEG was slower than the waking EEG, but it was not unitary. In fact, an entire set of different EEG patterns was observed during the same brief sleep period. The perspective now evolved to sleep being not only unique from wakefulness, but also being a dynamic, active state during which plenty is happening.

---

### Poetic Perspectives on Sleep

'Sleep, that knits up the
    ravell'd sleave of care,
The death of each day's life,
    sore labour's bath
Balm of hurt minds, great
    Nature's second course,
Chief nourisher in life's feast.'

WILLIAM SHAKESPEARE,
*MACBETH*

'Sleep is perverse as human
    nature,
Sleep is perverse as
    legislature...
So people who go to bed
    to sleep
Must count French premiers
    or sheep,
And people who ought to
    arise from bed
Yawn and go back to sleep
    instead.'

OGDEN NASH,
*READ THIS VIBRANT EXPOSÉ*

## SLEEP IS COMPOSED OF TWO FUNDAMENTALLY DIFFERENT STATES

It was another 17 years before the second paradigm shift occurred with the discovery of Rapid Eye Movement (REM) sleep in 1953. Now almost everyone is familiar with REM sleep, but 60 years ago, it lay undiscovered until a chance occurrence. A young graduate student named Eugene Aserinsky, studying at the University of Chicago under the sleep researcher Nathaniel Kleitman, had examined how children's attention lapsed when they momentarily closed their eyes, and the association between slow eye movement during sleep and the depth of sleep. Infants seemed a good vehicle to further examine how eye closure and eye movements contributed to sleep.

Infants tend to sleep a good deal following eye closure. During the experiment, Aserinsky observed that the electrodes he had applied to measure eye movements were recording some very erratic activity. Of course, anyone who has looked closely at a sleeping infant or toddler will be familiar with the eye movements that are detectable beneath closed eyelids. These observed movements were matched to an EEG pattern that was unique from anything else observed during sleep. The speed of the brain waves was very fast and resembled the EEG patterns observed

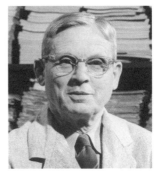

ABOVE *Nathaniel Kleitman of the University of Chicago was a pioneer in sleep research, and trained an entire generation of sleep researchers.*

RIGHT *Infants and toddlers spend a considerable portion of their sleep in Rapid Eye Movement (REM) sleep. These REMs can be easily observed beneath a child's closed eyelids.*

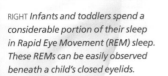

during active wakefulness. Thus, Rapid Eye Movement sleep was named and pronounced as a distinct state of consciousness. This was made even more intriguing by the soon-to-follow discovery from additional work studying adults, confirmed by another Kleitman student, William Dement, that dreaming emanated primarily from REM sleep. Following this exciting period in the science of sleep, it was safe to say that sleep comprised two active and fundamentally different states from those of wakefulness.

## SLEEP IS A HIGHLY REGULATED PROCESS

A good deal more was discovered about sleep over the next two decades. Like breathing or the beating of the heart, which we often take for granted, it turned out that sleep is actually a well-regulated process – when the sleep machinery is working properly, that is. When it is not, then sleep becomes highly 'dys-regulated'. Because we know how sleep is supposed to work, in subsequent chapters we will be able to identify those aspects of your sleep that may no longer be running smoothly.

## THE SLEEP CLOCK

Deep in the centre of the brain lies the tiny pineal gland, wherein resides a set of neurons called the suprachiasmatic nucleus (SCN). The SCN is the prime seat of control for a vast array of biological rhythms that occur every day, including the timing of sleep and wakefulness. The SCN has direct connections with the retinas in our eyes. This proves critical because, based on our exposure to the 24-hour, light–dark cycle, the SCN resets itself every day to keep the appropriate pace for our various daily rhythms. One of its tasks is to alert the pineal gland to increase the production and release of melatonin, a sleep-inducing hormone, at precisely the right time for us to make use of it.

**Light and the Sleep Cycle**

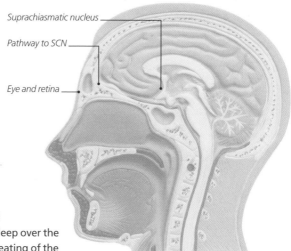

Suprachiasmatic nucleus

Pathway to SCN

Eye and retina

ABOVE *Light entrains the biological clock through pathways from the eye to the suprachiasmatic nucleus (SCN), which communicates with the pineal gland.*

## WHEN THE SLEEP CLOCK MALFUNCTIONS

To see how delicate the timing of sleep can be, you need only fly across multiple time zones and observe what happens to your sleep rhythm. Jet lag (and the poor sleep that accompanies it) is essentially the product of a confused SCN. Like a band with an inexperienced drummer, the jet-lagged brain and body struggle to get back on course. Conversely, a smoothly running sleep clock informs us when it's time for bed (and makes sure we're ready for it).

## THE SLEEP HOMEOSTAT

The sleep homeostat also regulates sleep. However, unlike the sleep clock, we cannot yet point to where this mechanism resides. We know that it works very much like a thermostat, though – alerting the boiler to start when it's too cold and to stop when it's warm enough. In this case the input to the sleep homeostat is the amount of wakefulness that has accumulated. When enough wakefulness has been accumulated, the sleep boiler fires up. As sleep burns off the accumulated wakefulness, the sleep boiler turns off and we wake with a full tank of alertness. While this may seem simplistic, mathematical models based on this concept can predict wake and sleep times with remarkable precision. We can also observe how the sleep homeostat works overtime to restore sleep homeostasis following sleep deprivation.

BELOW *The sleep clock is a delicate mechanism and can easily be knocked out of its natural routine when a person travels across several time zones.*

## A BROKEN HOMEOSTAT

If the sleep homeostat is 'broken', the sleep boiler may fail to turn on after the appropriate amount of wakefulness occurs. Or perhaps it helps to initiate sleep, but it takes a reading after about four hours and determines that it's time for the sleep boiler to shut down at 2.41 a.m. Being regularly awake for an hour or two, too late for any interesting television programme to be on and too early for you to reasonably start your day, is not the kind of consistency that a properly functioning homeostat should provide.

## THE REGULATORY SLEEP ENVIRONMENT

In addition to the sleep clock and sleep homeostat, there are several other components and systems involved in the regulation of sleep. These include an alphabet soup's worth of neurotransmitters and proteins, various cell assemblies, anatomical structures in the brainstem and the brain, and even substances produced by the immune system.

## WHAT SLEEP ACTUALLY IS

What is sleep then? Sleep is a state that is distinct from wakefulness, but not simply a unitary, quiescent state. Sleep is active, dynamic and organized. It is composed of the two completely different states of REM sleep and non-REM sleep. It is a highly and intricately regulated physiological process.

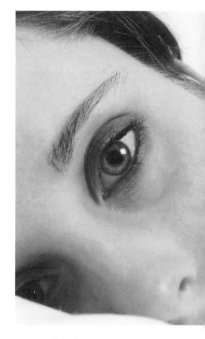

ABOVE *Wakefulness can occur at inappropriate times when the sleep homeostat is not functioning properly.*

LEFT *When the homeostatic drive for sleep exceeds the circadian alerting drive for wake, the stage is set for sleep to occur.*

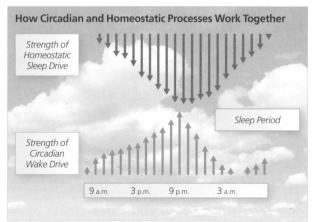

**How Circadian and Homeostatic Processes Work Together**

Strength of Homeostatic Sleep Drive

Sleep Period

Strength of Circadian Wake Drive

9 a.m.    3 p.m.    9 p.m.    3 a.m.

## WHAT HAPPENS WHEN WE SLEEP?

We have already established that sleep is a dynamic process in which the brain and body are each being rejuvenated while still performing vital functions. A variety of changes occur as we cycle back and forth between non-REM and REM sleep several times each night. Many of these changes can be monitored by polysomnography (PSG), the overnight measurement of physiological signals. These include electroencephalography (EEG) to measure brain-wave activity, as well as measurement of eye movements, facial muscle tone, heart rate, breathing, blood oxygen concentrations and leg movements. Other changes that occur during sleep can only be assessed via more intrusive methods, such as blood tests and brain imaging.

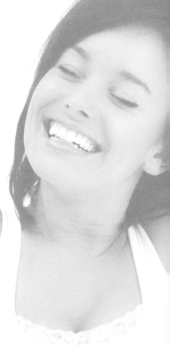

BELOW *Adequate amounts of good-quality sleep are needed to feel refreshed upon waking.*

### NON-REM SLEEP

Non-REM sleep is composed of three distinct stages of sleep, each defined by its unique EEG, eye movement and muscle-tone patterns. These stages are called Stage 1, Stage 2 and Stage 3 sleep. Until recently, Stage 4 was also recognized, but it was so similar to Stage 3 sleep that the two stages are usually now combined. The brain activity captured by EEGs is defined in terms of its speed in cycles per second (or Hertz [Hz]) and by the size of the individual brain waves (or amplitude).

## STAGE 1 SLEEP

As we close our eyes and prepare for sleep, the EEG pattern slows from its fast waking rhythm to a lower 8–13 Hz. As we enter sleep, the EEG is comprised of a mix of waves that are low in amplitude and are predominantly in the 4–7 Hz range, the eyes begin a slow rolling movement, and muscle tone relaxes somewhat. In its initial few minutes, Stage 1 sleep is very light. People may still be aware of environmental noises and have some active, though progressively disjointed, thoughts or visual images. If sleep is not interrupted here, Stage 1 serves as a brief five-minute transition between waking and Stage 2 sleep.

## STAGE 2 SLEEP

The transition to Stage 2 sleep is marked by the appearance of two novel EEG features, the sleep spindle and the K-complex. These occur over the backdrop of the 4–7 Hz low-amplitude EEG profile. Sleep spindles are dense bursts of EEG activity in the 12–14 Hz range that last between 0.5 and 1 second. The K-complex is a single EEG wave that is both slow (approximately 2 Hz) and high in amplitude. This stage may last 15–30 minutes: there are few, if any, eye movements and muscle tone is unchanged from Stage 1.

BELOW *Each state of consciousness and stage of sleep has a unique brain-activity pattern measured by electroencephalography (EEG).*

## STAGE 3 SLEEP

The transition to Stage 3 sleep occurs as slow wave activity (0.5–2.0 Hz) with high amplitude that begins to build during Stage 2. When any 30-second stretch of sleep contains at least 20 per cent of these slow waves, it is considered Stage 3 sleep. This stage, which is also known as slow-wave sleep, and more colloquially as deep sleep, may last 20–40 minutes. If depth of sleep is measured in terms of how difficult it is to arouse someone from sleep, this is the deepest part of sleep.

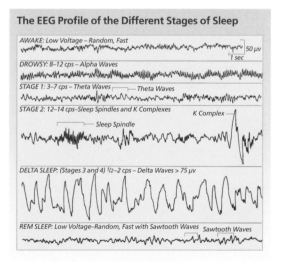

**The EEG Profile of the Different Stages of Sleep**

AWAKE: Low Voltage – Random, Fast
50 µv
1 sec

DROWSY: 8–12 cps – Alpha Waves

STAGE 1: 3–7 cps – Theta Waves ⌐— Theta Waves

STAGE 2: 12–14 cps–Sleep Spindles and K Complexes    K Complex —

⌐——— Sleep Spindle

DELTA SLEEP: (Stages 3 and 4) ¹/₂–2 cps – Delta Waves > 75 µv

REM SLEEP: Low Voltage–Random, Fast with Sawtooth Waves    Sawtooth Waves

## REM SLEEP

REM sleep occurs after approximately 80–90 minutes of sleep. The EEG profile in REM sleep is markedly different from that at any other time of sleep. It is random and fast (15–30 Hz), and except for some unique 'sawtooth waves', looks exactly like waking EEG. Muscle tone also decreases dramatically. Indeed, the entire body is in a state of semiparalysis. Of course, the most striking feature of REM sleep is the appearance of sharp eye movements to the left and right, as well as up and down. These REM sleep periods can last from as little as 5–10 minutes, to 30 minutes or more. As a graduate student, I was excited and amazed to be observing at first hand this utterly unique manifestation of an altered brain state the first time I observed these REMs on the computer screen. In retrospect, I became completely hooked on sleep medicine and sleep research that night.

## WHAT DO THE EYES SEE DURING RAPID EYE MOVEMENTS?

Given that the eyes are closed during sleep, the question arises as to whether the eye movements represent an internal scanning of dream imagery that may be present. This is an incredibly difficult question to answer, as it requires investigators to monitor eye movements on the computer screen, wake a research participant, and ask them what, if anything, they were dreaming about. Many such studies have been undertaken, with mixed results. Overall, the best that can be said is that recorded eye movements are associated with what is occurring during a dream some of the time.

### Active Ears During REM Sleep

Among the various sensory modalities available to us, visual sense occurs in nearly 100 per cent of reported dreams. Auditory sensation is the second most commonly reported sensation, occurring in approximately 65 per cent of dreams. Interestingly, mechanisms of hearing are active during REM sleep. Middle ear-muscle activity (or MEMA) is evoked by the first portion of loud sound bursts. Spontaneous MEMA seldom occurs outside of REM sleep. MEMA is somewhat associated with the presence of vivid auditory sensations of loud sounds in dreams.

BELOW *Signature eye movements of REM sleep are accompanied by more limited muscle activity than, but a similar EEG pattern to, waking.*

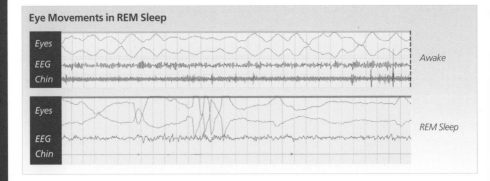

**Eye Movements in REM Sleep**

Eyes
EEG
Chin
*Awake*

Eyes
EEG
Chin
*REM Sleep*

## IF I NEVER DREAM, DO I HAVE ANY REM SLEEP?

Although there are always exceptions, the majority of us dream every night. Most of us simply do not remember our dreams. The inability to recall dreams, therefore, is certainly not an indication of REM sleep being completely absent.

## CYCLES OF SLEEP

Normal sleep is characterized by discrete episodes of non-REM and REM sleep that alternate several times during the night. Like so many biological processes, these cycles represent an ultradian rhythm that lasts approximately 90 minutes. As shown on page 25, sleep is well organized, progressing from Stage 1, 2 and 3 (non-REM sleep) to REM sleep. The majority of Stage 3 sleep occurs in the first half of the night, while the REM periods become increasingly longer as the night continues. Thus REM sleep tends to predominate in the second half of the night.

It is important to note that it is normal to wake, however briefly, during transitions to and from a REM period. Such awakenings are not always recalled. Repeated awakenings can be problematic, for at least two reasons. First, such awakenings disrupt the flow of sleep. Although it is possible to wake from Stage 3 sleep and return directly to Stage 3 sleep, it is more common for the brain and body to awaken and then go through Stage 1 and 2 sleep before returning to deeper sleep. As we will see, patients with sleep disorders such as sleep apnoea, who have dozens of brief awakenings per night, tend to have diminished amounts of Stage 3 sleep and REM sleep. In addition, readers with insomnia will know that even brief repeated awakenings become increasingly frustrating or discouraging, particularly when the experience is one of longer awakenings. Normal awakenings are to be expected, but should be brief in duration and few in number.

BELOW *A hypnogram provides a view of how we cycle through the stages of sleep several times each night.*

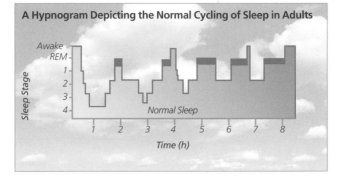

**A Hypnogram Depicting the Normal Cycling of Sleep in Adults**

Sleep Stage: Awake, REM, 1, 2, 3, 4

Normal Sleep

Time (h): 1 2 3 4 5 6 7 8

## BRAIN & BODY CHANGES DURING SLEEP

We now know that sleep is a dynamic state. Though many body functions slow down during sleep, many also have their own cycles, and others will make prolonged appearances.

## BASIC BODY FUNCTIONS DURING SLEEP

Heart rate, respiratory rate and blood pressure decrease during non-REM sleep, then fluctuate, become irregular, and can reach waking levels during active periods of REM sleep. Muscle tone decreases from waking levels during non-REM sleep and diminishes further while in REM sleep. There are brief muscle contractions throughout sleep, experienced as twitches or jerks. Men and women experience penile and clitoral erections during REM sleep. These are normal, but their function remains unexplained.

Although the normal body temperature is about 37°C (98.6°F), the actual average body temperature when taken under the tongue is 36.8°C (98.2°F). There is a fairly wide temperature range of 1.1°C (2.3°F) across the 24-hour day and these differences follow a unique rhythm. Temperature is highest during late morning and throughout the afternoon, begins to decrease in the early evening, and reaches its lowest point at about 4 a.m. before gradually increasing during the morning. For the average individual, sleep initiation coincides with a steep dip in body temperature; the low point is probably the time of night during REM sleep, when the discarded blanket is pulled back up.

Production of hormones, including cortisol, prolactin and thyroid hormones, follows a 24-hour rhythm, with evident differences between daytime and night-time production. Hormones secreted preferentially or almost exclusively during sleep include melatonin and the human growth hormone. Many substances involved in the immune system have their own daily production cycles, some of which peak during sleep.

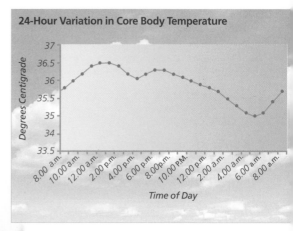

### 24-Hour Variation in Core Body Temperature

*Time of Day / Degrees Centigrade*

ABOVE *Core body temperature fluctuates throughout the day (and night).*

## BASIC BRAIN FUNCTIONS DURING SLEEP

Most processes in the human body are fully or partly controlled by the brain. It is possible to highlight features of sleep linked with changes in the brain, and we have seen how brain-wave activity changes throughout the course of the night.

Thinking is another exclusive brain activity. Most people can equate the onset of sleep with the cessation of thinking, but many will acknowledge that some form of thinking can persist into sleep. How useful this thinking is, however, is debatable. Some of us report being able to 'work through' a problem during sleep, but for most thinking becomes scattered and ceases. There is some evidence from experiments that thinking can occur into sleep, scenarios in which individuals were given auditory information and asked to respond by pressing a button near their dominant hand, or were woken up to report what they heard. In these experiments, button pushing can continue in the first few minutes of Stage 1 sleep, and individuals are able to identify some stimuli on waking, but memory is poorer than the simple motor responses. However, the longer experimenters waited to wake subjects, the less likely it was that the subjects could recall any information that was presented to them.

## THE SLEEPING BRAIN AND RESPONSIVENESS

As any parent knows, the sleeping brain is able to scan the environment for important stimuli and prompt an awakening at the first cry of a sick child. We wake more easily at the mention of our name than someone else's. Unfortunately, as any person with insomnia knows, the sleeping brain can also tune in to less important stimuli. Traffic noise, a neighbour's dog, a dripping tap, or a creak in the home can be seen as worthy of wakefulness. However, these stimuli have to be increasingly strong in the deeper stages of sleep in order to wake us.

Brain cells require energy, and their use of energy can be measured in terms of metabolic rates. There is less brain metabolism during sleep, but in REM sleep brain metabolism approaches that of the waking brain. REM sleep is so different from non-REM sleep that, depending on which sleep is occurring, numerous sites and neurochemicals in the brain have very different characteristics. This is so pronounced that some of these sites have been called 'REM-on' and 'REM-off' cells.

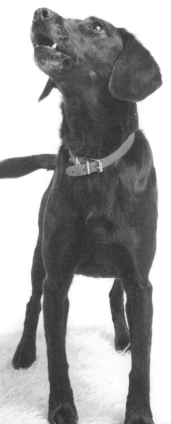

BELOW *The sleeping brain can still scan the environment for sounds and noises that demand its attention.*

# HOW MUCH SLEEP DO WE NEED?

Eight hours of sleep is the rule of thumb for adequate sleep; but is someone who sleeps nine hours per night getting too much, and is someone who gets seven hours per night getting too little? And is getting too little or too much sleep something that should concern us?

## SLEEP QUANTITY

The answer to these questions depends on how sleep quantity (or sleep duration) is measured. In large surveys of people's average sleep duration in Britain and the United States, answers varied widely. Around 30 per cent reported sleeping more than eight hours per night and 15 per cent reported sleeping less than six hours. Several such surveys have been conducted, and the overall average has consistently come in around seven hours per night. So, perhaps the average sleep duration is not eight, but seven hours per night.

In other surveys in which large samples of adults were asked to distinguish between average sleep duration during weekdays compared with weekends, the weekday averages again were about seven hours per night. Their average weekend sleep duration was approximately eight hours, presumably 'catching up' on lost sleep during the standard work week.

## AVERAGE SLEEP NEED

The last chapter in the sleep-duration story revolves around determining precisely the average sleep need (as opposed to the sleep that is reported). In order to do this, investigators recruited subjects to have their sleep recorded for several consecutive nights, allowing them to sleep for as long as they could. First, when given the opportunity to sleep more than their reported sleep duration, the participants took full advantage. Then, once sleep stabilized, the average amount of sleep achieved was approximately eight hours, six minutes. So, we seem to have come full circle back to the eight-hour-per-night rule of thumb (as an average).

**Other Perspectives on Sleep Quantity**

'The day and night consist of 24 hours. It is sufficient for a person to sleep a third thereof…'

MAIMONIDES

'The amount of sleep required by the average person is five minutes more.'

WILSON MIZENER

'Without enough sleep, we all become tall two-year-olds.'

JOJO JENSEN, *DIRT FARMER WISDOM*, 2002

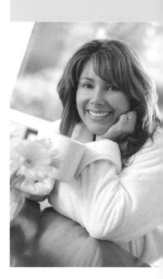

ABOVE *Feeling refreshed after a night's sleep requires both an adequate amount of sleep and good-quality sleep.*

## SLEEP QUALITY

Eight hours of good sleep feels different from eight hours of poor sleep. Good-quality sleep is largely uninterrupted, allowing the brain and body to cycle through all stages of sleep three, four, even five times per night. When this occurs, we are able to achieve refreshing sleep, which is found in Stage 3 sleep (slow-wave sleep) and REM sleep. Sleep researchers question whether Stage 1 sleep has any useful function other than being a transitional stage between wakefulness and deeper stages of sleep. Even Stage 2 sleep is thought to pale in comparison to the benefits of slow-wave sleep, which comprises 60–80 minutes of an eight-hour sleep period in normal young to middle-aged adults. REM sleep typically comprises 80–100 minutes.

If slow-wave sleep and REM sleep are the good stuff, it seems inefficient to bother with the other stages of sleep. There seems to be no ready solution to this. Stage 1 and Stage 2 sleep are the gateway to slow-wave and to REM sleep.

## SHORT SLEEPERS

Some rare individuals, called 'short sleepers', naturally sleep two to three fewer hours than others and still feel refreshed. Part of their solution is that they pack higher percentages of slow-wave sleep, and to a lesser extent REM sleep, into those five to six hours than normal sleepers do. The search for a way to achieve this in normal sleepers has proved elusive. Therefore, for most of us the key to good-quality sleep is to give ourselves the opportunity to get our individual required sleep duration, and to do so without being interrupted by more than a few normal brief awakenings.

RIGHT *The category denoted by 3 hours includes persons who reported sleeping anywhere from 3 hours to 3 hours and 59 minutes, the category denoted by 4 hours includes times from 4 hours to 4 hours and 59 minutes, and so on.*

### Am I Getting What I Need?

If you have a sleep disorder, try recalling a period in your adult life when you were getting good sleep and estimate your average sleep duration. If you are a normal sleeper, go to bed at a regular time, sleep for as long as you can, and note how long you sleep. Avoid napping during the day, but if you do, count it in your total sleep time the next night. Repeat each night until you feel rested on waking and the total nightly sleep time has evened out. This is your individual sleep need. It is impossible to know what amounts of slow-wave sleep and REM sleep are normal for you unless you do this exercise while wearing sleep-recording equipment.

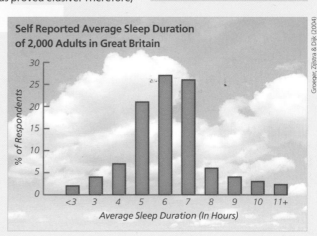

**Self Reported Average Sleep Duration of 2,000 Adults in Great Britain**

Groeger, Zijlstra & Dijk (2004)

# WHAT IS THE FUNCTION OF SLEEP?

The need for sleep is universal, extending to all mammals, birds and some reptiles. Certainly for humans, sleep is a basic need. Sleep deprivation propels us to pursue sleep as we would pursue water across a desert. Although we understand that food and water are required for the body to function, it is more difficult to fathom *why* we actually need to sleep. This leads us to explore the function of sleep.

### ENERGY CONSERVATION

It is well known that the rate of metabolism diminishes during sleep. One function of sleep, therefore, is thought to be the conservation of energy. In addition, most of the major organs are less active during sleep, ostensibly providing for less wear and tear than if they were equally active across the 24-hour day.

### LEARNING & MEMORY

Despite the conservation of energy that occurs during sleep, some processes are actually elevated. In 2006, researchers from Brigham and Women's Hospital, University of Pennsylvania, and Harvard Medical School conducted a study of 33 women and 27 men aged between 18 and 39.

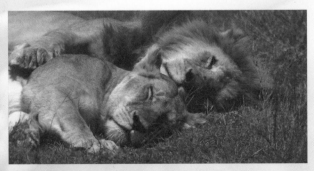

LEFT *Sleep is a great restorative, and essential to all mammals, birds and some reptiles.*

In this experiment, they gave the participants sets of paired words to memorize and then tested their recall after a full night's sleep and after a night of inadequate sleep. They found that sleep 'plays an active role in memory consolidation' and that sleep-deprivation and 'cramming' the night before an exam is counterproductive.

## SLEEP & LEARNING

The advice to get a good night's sleep before a big exam is well founded. Several research studies in both animals and humans point to an exquisite role of sleep to enhance recall of recently learned material. Although these points continue to be debated and investigated, the neuronal activity that occurs in sleep is believed to clear out neuronal pathways that contain unnecessary information, and rehearses the neuronal connections and pathways containing new information. It seems that a critical function of sleep is to promote the consolidation of new learning into long-term memory.

## DREAMING & REM SLEEP

Sleep, of course, allows REM sleep and dreaming to occur. The function of REM sleep is associated with brain development in infants and with the memory-consolidation process in adults. REM sleep also enables dreaming to take place, which can be important for emotional regulation (and as a source of interesting party conversation).

## HOW DOES REMOVING SLEEP IMPAIR US?

Sleep deprivation can diminish the production of growth hormones and disturb learning and memory. Over a relatively short time (a week), the effects of nightly partial sleep deprivation lead to decreases in performance on cognitive and motor tasks equivalent to decrements observed in persons with blood alcohol contents of 0.10 per cent (above the legal limit, for example, in the United Kingdom and the United States). At the extreme, prolonged total sleep deprivation in laboratory rats leads to a breakdown in their ability to combat infection, to an inability to regulate body temperature, and to death in a matter of weeks. Although this may seem dramatic, there is much evidence to support the notion that sleep is vital to life.

### Repair & Regeneration

Sleep provides the time and conditions for several restorative body processes to take place. Proteins, cells and tissue are synthesized in greater amounts during sleep than during wakefulness. Production and release of hormones, including human growth hormone (HGH), also occurs during sleep. When children are deprived of sleep, their growth rate is blunted by a diminished release of growth hormone.

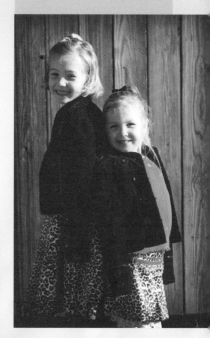

# DREAMS & DREAMING

Dreaming is an intriguing component of our sleep lives. REM sleep, which is intimately associated with dreaming, is an odd form of sleep and from an evolutionary perspective is equally odd in that it has poor survival value. It utilizes a lot of energy, promotes wear and tear on neurons and renders the individual vulnerable to attack with its paralysis like muscle tone and diminished vigilance. One logical deduction is that REM sleep evolved in all mammals despite these encumbrances because it allows dreaming to occur. By extension, therefore, dreaming must be important. Whether dreams themselves are important is more controversial.

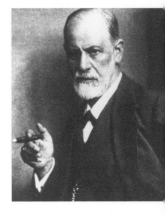

ABOVE *In the early twentieth century, neurologist Sigmund Freud emphasized the importance of dreams in his psychoanalytic theory.*

BELOW *REM sleep engages parts of the brain that are more dormant during other stages of sleep.*

**Engaged Areas of the Brain During REM Sleep**

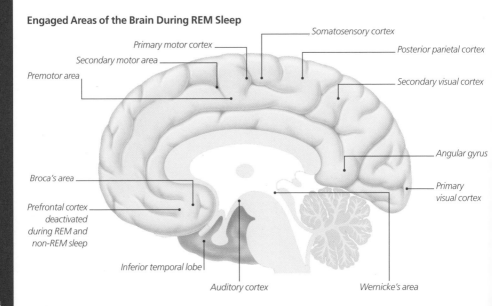

Primary motor cortex

Secondary motor area

Premotor area

Somatosensory cortex

Posterior parietal cortex

Secondary visual cortex

Angular gyrus

Broca's area

Prefrontal cortex deactivated during REM and non-REM sleep

Primary visual cortex

Inferior temporal lobe

Auditory cortex

Wernicke's area

## A BRIEF HISTORY OF DREAMS

Dreams have been linked with prophecies and healing throughout the ages. Followers of Asclepius, the Greek god of medicine, built healing temples called *asclepieion*, where patients reported dreams to priests in order to aid diagnosis and treatment. In modern times, Austrian neurologist Sigmund Freud and Swiss psychiatrist Carl Jung further popularized the importance of dreams. In the 1960s and 1970s, the discovery of REM sleep and its link to dreaming led to a flurry of dream research and refinements.

## SOME THINGS WE KNOW ABOUT DREAMS

In REM and non-REM sleep, there are periods of dreaming and non-dreaming. Some have argued whether non-REM dreams are dreams. REM dreams tend to be longer and more frequent, vivid, dramatic, emotional, perceptual and bizarre than non-REM dreams; non-REM dreams are more thoughtlike and conceptual.

## THE NEUROBIOLOGY OF DREAMING

The portions of the brain that are active or inactive in REM sleep can be connected to the way dreams are formed. First, the fast-frequency brain activity that occurs in REM sleep is associated with cognitive activities that occur during wakefulness. Second, there are increased bursts of electrical activity from the brainstem in REM sleep, and these are associated with eye movements. Third, several areas of the brain involved in emotion and memory become reactivated in REM sleep after being dormant during non-REM sleep. Fourth, the prefrontal cortex, which performs executive functions during wakefulness, remains deactivated during non-REM and REM sleep, and a host of neurochemicals change their balance during REM sleep to promote dreaming, including access to various types of memories and emotions. These neurochemicals also enable critical thinking to be suspended, thus allowing unlikely scenes, which would be impossible in waking life, to proceed without question. These are very satisfying discoveries for sleep researchers, but provide little in terms of an explanation for why dreaming occurs and what dreams mean.

### The Function of Dreaming

Some researchers say dreaming is a purely biological function, maintaining neural networks at an optimum level. Variations of this idea discount dreams as the brain weaving the cacophony of REM-sleep stimulation into a quasi-plausible storyline. Others say dreaming occurs to guide, heal, solve problems, or regulate emotion. Most agree dreaming is important. When REM sleep is curtailed for one or more nights, there is a REM-sleep rebound that exceeds normal levels, and dreams are longer and more intense. Most also agree that dreams can be a synthesis of random material, devoid of any meaning, or meaningful for the individual.

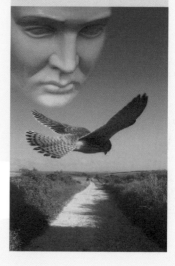

## COMMON DREAMS

Despite the bizarre nature of some dreams, the majority of dreams are not bizarre – their story lines are coherent, and they would be credible if described as a waking event. Daily hassles, problems and life stressors are often the subject of dreams. Several research studies note that daily stressors, such as health problems, academic stress and occupational concerns, are incorporated into dreams, and that the more severe the stressor, the more often it appears in dreams.

## UNCOMMON DREAMS

Recurrent dreams tend to be more negative than non-recurring dreams, and they also tend to be activated by stress. For instance, young adults several years out of school will attest to having their typical stress dream during a new period of life stress. Such dreams involve something like showing up for final exams realizing that they had forgotten to attend classes all year, and then realizing that they had shown up in their underwear. Following severe stress, dreams are especially negative and can be considered nightmares.

BELOW RIGHT *Lucid dreamers realize they are dreaming, and can consciously alter their dreams (perhaps deciding to test out some dream flight).*

Much has been made of famous examples of creative dreams in both the arts and sciences. Composers such as Mozart, Beethoven and Wagner said that some of their works were inspired by dreams. Tartini, an Italian composer, reported transposing an entire violin sonata that the Devil was playing in his dream. The plot for *Dr Jekyll and Mr Hyde* came to Robert Louis Stevenson during sleep, and Samuel Taylor Coleridge dreamed about 200 lines of *Kubla Khan* (albeit that may have been opium-inspired). From the sciences, Elias Howe's invention of the sewing machine and Friedrich Kekulé's discovery of the

### A Sample of Common Dream Themes in College Students

| Rank | Theme | % of Dreams |
|------|-------|-------------|
| 1 | Being chased, but not hurt | 78 |
| 2 | Sexual experiences | 77 |
| 3 | School, teachers, studying | 72 |
| 4 | Falling | 72 |
| 5 | Arriving too late | 65 |
| 6 | Trying repeatedly to do something | 61 |
| 7 | Being on the verge of falling | 58 |
| 8 | A person now alive is dead | 53 |
| 9 | Flying or soaring | 50 |
| 10 | Failing an exam | 49 |
| 11 | Being frozen with fright | 49 |
| 12 | Being physically attacked | 48 |
| 13 | A person now dead is alive | 45 |
| 14 | Sensing a presence in the room | 44 |
| 15 | Being naked | 40 |

*Adapted from Zadraand & Nielsen (1999)*

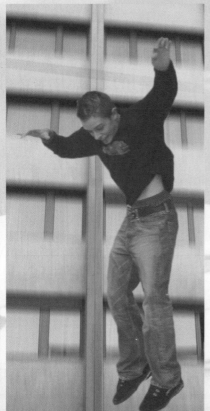

atomic structure of benzene came from dreams. Otto Loewi's experimental design that led to the discovery of the first neurotransmitter and the 1936 Nobel Prize came to him during sleep. There are doubtless other instances of dreams directly and indirectly sparking ideas and creations, great and small.

## LUCID DREAMING

Lucid dreaming is an uncommon experience. This phenomenon occurs when dreamers become aware that they are dreaming. This consciousness is called 'lucidity'. Often, when dreamers become lucid, they immediately wake up. Some individuals, however, can continue to dream and maintain their lucidity, enabling them to then consciously manipulate their dream. In essence, they become the directors of their own dream films. Very experienced lucid dreamers studied in the sleep-research lab have even been able to signal to the researchers when they become lucid through a prearranged series of eye movements. Although consistent lucid dreaming is uncommon, lucid dreaming can be learned through practice (interested readers are directed to Stephen LaBerges' informative book, *Lucid Dreaming*).

## A MOOD-REGULATING ROLE OF DREAMING

In closing this section on dreams, I offer one middle-of-the-road approach to dreaming espoused by Rosalind Cartwright, a long-time sleep researcher. She contends that dreaming is a mood-regulating system, noting first that dream content is related to daytime emotional events and that dreams are most salient after such events. Next, she points to research showing that a negative mood present at sleep onset is diminished by morning when dreaming is allowed to occur. Finally, she has shown that subjects who dream about a troubling life event are less likely to be depressed at a later time than those who do not dream about the event. Although these data do not fully support a mood-regulating function of dreaming, they do give the notion some credence.

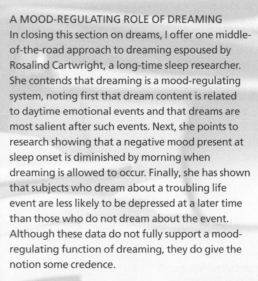

## SLEEP THROUGHOUT THE LIFESPAN

Sleep duration, sleep quality and patterns of sleep change dramatically across the entire lifespan. The most pronounced changes occur during infancy, childhood and adolescence, and represent normal developmental changes. In adulthood, there is a more gradual change in sleep that is normal and age-related. Most changes in sleep during adulthood are not necessarily normal developmental changes, but are the indirect result of changes in health and more direct changes because of sleep disorders.

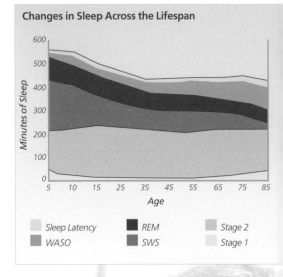

### SLEEP IN INFANTS & CHILDREN

Young infants sleep approximately two-thirds of a 24-hour day, with approximately eight hours a day spent in REM sleep. Total sleep remains fairly stable over the first year of life, although sleep becomes gradually more consolidated during night-time hours and REM sleep decreases to three to four hours per day. From about 18–24 months, total sleep time gradually decreases to about 10–12 hours in six- to ten-year-olds, while the percentage of sleep time spent in REM sleep decreases to the 20–25 per cent level observed in adults.

By five to six years of age, sleep is well organized into the sleep-stage patterns. The largest changes that occur during the ages of five to ten years is that naps become rare and slow-wave sleep time decreases from approximately two hours to 70–90 minutes.

ABOVE *Total sleep time does not vary much with age through most of adulthood, although slow-wave sleep does diminish (after Ohayon, Carskadon, Guilleminault et al., 2004).*

RIGHT *Inadequate sleep duration in adolescents is associated with increased daytime sleepiness.*

## SLEEP IN ADOLESCENTS

Adolescents need similar amounts of sleep to children and more than adults. They are notorious for getting too little sleep during the week and trying to make up for it on weekends, partly because of changes in their circadian rhythms and the demands of the school system. The adolescent sleep clock gets set to a later bedtime. This makes it difficult to fall asleep early enough to get the nine hours of sleep that average teenagers require.

## SLEEP IN ADULTHOOD

In early adulthood, total sleep time decreases to about eight hours and remains fairly constant through life. There is a gradual reduction in slow-wave sleep, which can be absent by age 60 or earlier (with a corresponding increase in Stage 2 sleep). This occurs earlier in men than in women, and is believed to be related to age-related declines in neurons and their interconnectivity. Healthy older adults retain slow-wave sleep into later life.

## DISTURBANCES TO SLEEP AS WE AGE

Most medical conditions, chronic and long-lasting or acute and temporary, alter sleep. Many medications alter the structure of sleep, by increasing or decreasing REM sleep (and, to a lesser extent, slow-wave sleep). Medication side effects often include insomnia or drowsiness. Finally, rates of sleep disorders, such as sleep apnoea, insomnia and restless leg syndrome, increase with age and alter sleep duration, quality and structure.

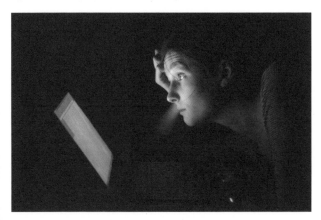

### Sleep Storm – Male Version

Imagine a middle-aged man with a history of off-and-on low back pain; the pain is not resolving as it has in the past. He cannot find a comfortable position to sleep, experiences awakenings and wakes unrefreshed. He continues to work, but cuts back on his already inconsistent exercise. He puts on a few pounds and his family begins to complain about his snoring. His blood pressure is elevated; he feels depressed and wiped out most of the day. What's going on?

Most pain conditions disrupt sleep. Poor sleep exacerbates sensitivity, which worsens sleep (vicious cycle 1). Snoring is linked to weight gain: he now has mild sleep apnoea, interrupting his sleep further. The apnoea increases daytime fatigue and sleepiness, diminishing physical activity, leading to more weight gain and worse apnoea (vicious cycle 2). The link between depression and insomnia is vicious cycle 3; cycles 4, 5 and 6 could begin if he starts taking pain, anti-depressant or blood-pressure medications. However, all these cycles are reversible using the programme in this book.

## SLEEP CHANGES IN WOMEN

Several experiences unique to women can alter their sleep, but research in these areas is limited, and can be complicated to implement. Women have reported poorer sleep premenstrually. Some, but not all, laboratory sleep studies have corroborated this.

## PREGNANCY & THE MENOPAUSE

Pregnancy is associated with an increased number of awakenings and lower total sleep time, with some indications that slow-wave sleep is diminished. Increased sleepiness occurs more often in the first trimester, whereas insomnia symptoms occur more regularly in the third trimester. In addition, pregnant women can develop snoring and some sleep-disordered breathing, as well as restless leg syndrome; all tend to abate postpartum. The postpartum period, however, is a time of disrupted sleep due to hormonal changes taking place and the infant's sleep cycle. In peri- and postmenopause, hot flushes disrupt sleep. Insomnia is the most commonly reported problem and thought to be related primarily to nocturnal hot flushes. Insomnia is more prevalent in women than in men. This may be partly because of the unique biological stressors and life events that women experience.

### Sleep Storm – Female Version

Imagine a woman after her third pregnancy, still depressed after her postpartum period, and her sleep has not returned to normal. It takes hours to fall asleep. She is not losing weight, despite her same vegetarian diet and returning to work. She has started to snore and her legs are uncomfortable during the day and jittery at night. Her physician says she is anaemic. What is going on? Insomnia developed during pregnancy is fuelled by restless leg syndrome, probably due to low iron in her diet, a potential breathing-related sleep disorder caused by her weight, and insomnia linked with depression. Diet and weight management may reverse the first two factors. The insomnia can then be addressed, even in the face of mild depression, (more severe depression may require its own treatment).

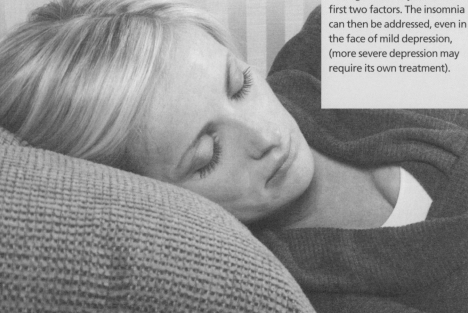

## IS INSOMNIA INEVITABLE?

For the vast majority of us insomnia is inevitable. That is only because most of us will suffer at least one, if not several, brief bouts of insomnia that may last a week or two in the midst of some life stressor. Chronic insomnia that persists for months and years, however, is far from inevitable. To be sure, the rates of insomnia do increase with age but the majority of adults do not develop chronic insomnia. Moreover, once insomnia does become problematic, there are several very effective ways to treat it, cure it and keep it at bay. While there are people who report that they have suffered through insomnia for years, that does not need to be you, and you can win this battle by using the strategies found in this book.

### Older Adults Do Not Need Less Sleep

It is important to dispel the myth that older adults require less sleep. Our sleep needs remain constant throughout our adult lives. Older adults may begin to alter their sleep schedule in a way that leads to less sleep, or they may develop sleep disorders that curtail their sleep. For example, the occasional weekend nap may turn into a daily afternoon nap during full retirement. The 20-minute catnap for an older person can be restorative, but a daily two-hour nap is a recipe for disrupting the sleep clock and may lead to overall loss of sleep. Alternatively, older adults taking several medications may find themselves on pills that make them sleepy during the day and cause insomnia at night. They may sleep less than they used to, but this is a problem to be solved and not the normal development of sleep in later years. A healthy 82-year-old who felt great on 7.5 hours of sleep per night at age 52 still needs 7.5 hours a night of sleep to function optimally.

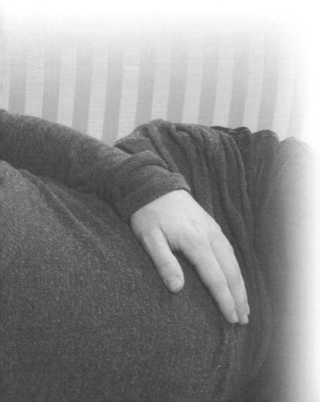

LEFT *The rate of insomnia tends to increase with age, especially for women.*

There are more than 100 recognized sleep disorders in the International Classification of Sleep Disorders. We will cover the more common of these sleep disorders, and a few less common ones, in this chapter. Although we are mainly interested in insomnia, the high occurrence of these other sleep disorders is reason enough to be aware of them. Beyond this, however, these disorders can sometimes occur along with insomnia, may themselves cause or worsen insomnia, or may mimic what we think is insomnia.

# CHAPTER 2
# IDENTIFYING SLEEP DISORDERS

## SLEEP-RELATED BREATHING DISORDERS

A number of overlapping and distinct sleep disorders involve breathing problems that occur during sleep. These include snoring, obstructive sleep apnoea, upper-airway resistance syndrome, central sleep apnoea and hypoventilation syndromes. Most of these conditions disturb sleep in one or more ways. They are fairly common in adults but less common in children. All of these disorders are in some way related to physiological factors that are congenital, appear over time or are due to a co-occurring medical condition. Most of these disorders respond well to the available treatments.

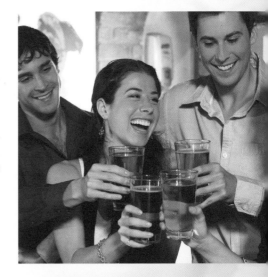

BELOW *Alcohol in moderate amounts is enjoyable, but it is also a muscle relaxant and can cause or exacerbate a snoring problem.*

### SNORING

Snoring is a very common condition that occurs in one-quarter to one-third of adults and approximately 10 per cent of children. It also tends to increase with age. Snoring occurs primarily during inhalation and seldom during exhalation. It occurs when air flow from the mouth and nose on its way to the lungs is restricted in some manner. The noise of snoring is produced by the vibration of tissue in the back of the throat as air moves across it. The sound originates in the back of the throat, though it may sound as if it comes from the nose, mouth or both. Snoring can occur in any stage of sleep, although it tends to be worse in slow-wave sleep and REM sleep.

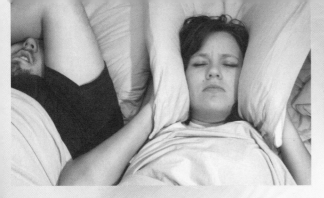

## WHAT CAUSES SNORING?

Anything that restricts airflow may cause snoring. Some people may simply have very narrow airways. Others may have large tongues, uvulas (the flap of skin that hangs down at the back of the throat) or tonsils. Tonsils can be a primary cause of snoring in children. Obstructions in the nasal passages, which could be caused by a deviated septum or the growth of nasal polyps, would also restrict airflow and produce snoring.

Many readers will no doubt have had the experience of snoring during colds. A stuffy nose caused by colds, allergies or the occasional raisin deposited in a nostril by a child, can all cause temporary snoring.

## IS SNORING BAD FOR ME (OR JUST FOR THOSE AROUND ME)?

At the very least, snoring is disruptive to the sleep of those around the snorer. Such persons are the best judges of the frequency and loudness of snoring. Some people report dry mouths or sore throats related to snoring. For many people, snoring may have no negative impact on their health. Loud snoring may disrupt your sleep by causing brief arousals and full awakenings. If you snore, but feel rested upon awakening and do not experience fatigue or sleepiness during the day, then the snoring may be completely benign (not counting the irritation it may cause your bed partner). Some researchers believe that snoring may be a precursor to the development of obstructive sleep apnoea (see page 48). Although this is not proven, it is the case that approximately 50 per cent of people who snore loudly also have obstructive sleep apnoea. People who snore have a higher rate of heart disease, which is a leading cause of death in industrialized nations.

### More Causes of Snoring

Although it sounds a bit silly, sleep itself can cause snoring. You will recall that muscle tone decreases during sleep. The tautness of the airway is maintained by a number of muscles, which relax during sleep. This explains why a person quietly resting on a sofa will not snore when awake, but begins to snore on falling asleep.

Snoring is more common in people who are overweight. Weight gain leads to an increase in fatty tissue in the back of the throat, essentially reducing the size of the airway. This is the main reason that snoring can develop during pregnancy. Smoking, alcohol and some medications (particularly those that have muscle-relaxing properties) also increase the risk of snoring. Given this lengthy list of causes, it is no wonder that snoring is so prevalent.

## WHAT CAN BE DONE ABOUT SNORING?

If you are concerned about your snoring, the best place to start is to see a sleep specialist. The consultation may be followed by an overnight sleep study to determine if, and how, the snoring is disrupting your sleep. There are now sleep centres within driving proximity in most areas of the United Kingdom. Make sure that such centres are recognised by the British Sleep Society or check with your doctor.

A number of proven treatments for snoring exist. Some simple approaches warrant attention. People who started snoring after gaining weight will want to give weight loss a try. If the relationship between weight gain and the beginning of snoring is unknown, but the individual is overweight, then weight loss should again be considered. Avoiding evening alcohol use and medications that may decrease muscle tone should also be considered. Persons with persistently stuffy noses can ask their GP about nasal sprays that may keep their nasal passages clear at night. Finally, people who snore primarily when sleeping on their backs may benefit from learning to sleep exclusively on their sides.

### Treatment of Sleep Disorders

More information about the treatment of sleep disorders may be gathered from the British Sleep Society, which is a professional organisation and registered British charity. Check their website at: *http://www.sleeping.org.uk*

BELOW *Snoring tends to be worse when sleeping in the supine position (on your back).*

### Supine Position

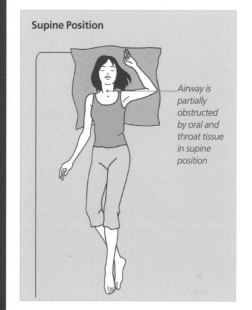

Airway is partially obstructed by oral and throat tissue in supine position

### Side Position

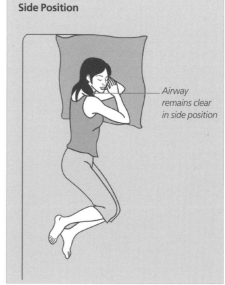

Airway remains clear in side position

More involved treatments include various types of oral appliances that are worn to maintain adequate amounts of airflow during the night. These appliances are essentially a version of a mouth guard or retainer that either keeps the tongue or the entire jaw in a more forward position than normally occurs during sleep.

MORE TREATMENTS FOR SNORING

A variety of surgical procedures can also be undertaken to remove or decrease the amount of tissue that may be restricting airflow. These can include removal of the tonsils, nasal surgery to correct deformations or remove polyps, or removal or reduction of the uvula or parts of the soft palate. A sleep specialist can advise you about surgical options, which are typically performed in an outpatient setting by ear, nose and throat specialists.

One treatment that is extensively used for obstructive sleep apnoea can be helpful for snoring when sleep apnoea is also present. Continuous positive airway pressure (CPAP) is very effective for this. We will discuss this treatment more fully in the section on obstructive sleep apnoea (see page 54).

Products that are marketed specifically for snoring, such as nasal or throat sprays, or some nasal strips, have been subjected to little research to determine their effectiveness in reducing snoring. Other alternative approaches have no supporting research and no real basis for why they would be effective. These include things like hypnosis, antisnoring CDs, magnets, homoeopathic remedies and natural products. One approach that might warrant a closer look, as it at least has some theoretical basis for having an effect on snoring and some limited research support, is to perform muscle-strengthening exercises that target the airway.

## Positional Therapy

If you snore primarily on your back, you can avoid repeated poking and prodding from your bed partner by employing the 'tennis-ball trick'. Place a tennis ball or rolled-up sock in the pocket of a T-shirt or pyjama top and wear it back to front (or sew it into the middle of the back of the garment). When you roll onto your back you will turn back to your side. Alternatives of this theme include using a thick pillow or foam wedge to keep yourself in a side position. There are even position alarms that can be worn to alert you to move to your side.

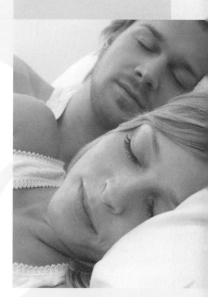

RIGHT *Learning to sleep on your side will help to prevent snoring and encourage peaceful sleep.*

## OBSTRUCTIVE SLEEP APNOEA

Obstructive sleep apnoea (OSA) is a sleep-related breathing disorder that causes breathing to be briefly and repeatedly stopped or reduced during sleep. Apnoea is the term used to describe a cessation of breathing that lasts for at least ten seconds during sleep. The apnoea occurs when the airway essentially collapses and completely closes off the passageway. When this happens, the tongue can fall back into the throat a little and further block the airway.

## WHAT HAPPENS DURING SLEEP APNOEA

During apnoea, the lung and its musculature continue to attempt to breathe and the chest and abdomen continue to move, and oxygen levels in the bloodstream begin to drop as no new oxygen enters the lungs. Meanwhile, carbon-dioxide levels begin to rise, as the lungs are unable to expel old air. Our bodies contain a number of receptors that keep track of carbon dioxide levels and send a distress signal to the brain. When the brain receives the signal, it orders the body to do something to end the apnoea. That something comes in the form of a snort or gasp to clear the airway, often accompanied by a brief arousal of a few seconds. With the crisis averted, normal breathing resumes and the brain quickly returns to sleep. This process can occur 100 or more times per night. Interestingly, young infants exhibit a natural apnoea as they automatically hold their breath underwater; the epiglottis closes over in response to submersion, and the heart rate slows.

### The Sights & Sounds of OSA

Snoring frequently, though not always, accompanies OSA. Observing someone with sleep apnoea who snores can be somewhat alarming. The steady snore suddenly stops. There is a pronounced silence. And no breathing … for ten seconds … no breathing … chest movement becomes more insistent, but still no breathing … 15 seconds … 20 seconds … then a loud snort, a sudden body movement and a deep breath. Some normal breaths. Commence snoring. Repeat. The first time I saw this occur repeatedly in a patient, my insightful thought was 'that cannot be good for you'.

## HOW APNOEA APPEARS WHEN MONITORED

On a computer screen, a host of lines show physiological activity. Prior to apnoea, there are normal EEG patterns for Stage 2 sleep – regularly recurring sinusoidal lines depicting air inflow and outflow, abdominal and upper chest movement; a line depicting bursts of snoring; a steady line showing oxygen saturation levels in the bloodstream of 97–100 per cent; and a normal heart rhythm from an EKG tracing (electrocardiogram). At the onset of apnoea, the EEG shows continued Stage 2 sleep, the snore line is quiet, airflow flatlines, chest and abdominal effort diminishes and oxygen saturation creeps downward. As apnoea progresses, the EKG shows an increase in heart rate (though decreases also occur). Oxygen saturations may remain stable at 2–4 per cent below their normal levels or may drop to levels around 70 per cent and lower.

When apnoea ends, the snore channel records a burst, EEGs show a brief arousal, movement is recorded in muscle-activity signals, and airflow and breathing effort produce large  waves, which return to normal after a breath or two, and heart rate and oxygen saturation return to their normal levels.

BELOW *A quiet, undisturbed sleep requires air to pass unrestricted through the mouth and down the windpipe into the lungs.*

**Passage of Air from Mouth to Lungs**

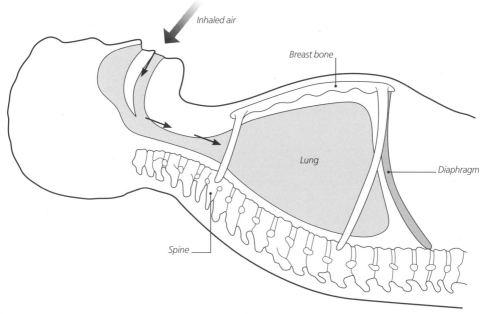

Inhaled air

Breast bone

Lung

Diaphragm

Spine

## Hypopnoeas Interspersed with Normal Breathing

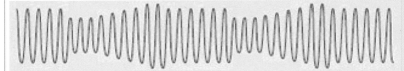

WHAT IS AN HYPOPNOEA?

An hypopnoea is a partial closure of the airway. As with apnoea, hypopnoea may be preceded by snoring and end with a snort or gasp, though the latter is less common or less pronounced than with apnoea. When recorded in a sleep lab, the various physiological changes are less pronounced than those seen with apnoea. There is a reduction in airflow that lasts for at least ten seconds and is associated with a modest decrease in oxygen saturation and/or is followed by an EEG arousal. Persons with OSA have both apnoeas and hypopnoeas, and the mix can vary. Although examples here refer to apnoeas occurring during Stage 2 sleep, apnoeas and hypopnoeas can occur in any stage of sleep. In fact, because of increased loss of muscle tone during REM sleep, apnoeas are longer, and more severe, in REM sleep.

WHAT IS UPPER-AIRWAY RESISTANCE SYNDROME?

Upper-airway resistance syndrome (UARS) is currently categorized as a mild form of OSA. The breathing events that gave rise to the recognition of UARS are smaller than hypopnoeas. They are called respiratory effort-related arousals because there is a very modest decrease in airflow and increase in breathing effort, followed by an arousal captured on the EEG.

THE PREVALENCE OF OSA

Most specialists agree that at least 4 per cent of men and 2 per cent of women have OSA. OSA may occur in any adult age group, although it is increasingly common between middle and old age. The highest prevalence is between the ages of 40–65. OSA severity worsens over time when left untreated. Conservative estimates state 2 per cent of healthy children have OSA. Up to 10–20 per cent of children who are habitual snorers have OSA.

ABOVE *An hypopnoea occurs when the airway partially closes and results in decreased airflow.*

## THE CAUSES OF OSA

Causes of OSA closely mirror those of snoring, and include all manner of physical characteristics or conditions that restrict airflow by reducing the size of the airway. This includes stuffy noses, large tonsils, tongues and uvulas. Narrow airways sometimes occur because of genes or as part of another genetic condition. For instance, children and adults with Down syndrome have higher levels of OSA because of the size of their tongues, small oral cavity and overall reduced muscle tone.

By far the most common cause of OSA is being overweight. The Body Mass Index (BMI) is a quick way to determine whether you are overweight for your height. It produces a figure that ranges from about 15 to 40 and above, where a BMI of 25 and above is considered overweight. Men and women with a BMI over 27 have twice the rates of snoring and OSA than do those with a BMI under 27. There are large individual variances in the relationship between BMI and OSA. To begin with, each of us has a different threshold above which we are likely to develop OSA. For some of us, it can develop as soon as we are ten pounds overweight and for others that threshold may be at a 100 pounds overweight. Still others develop apnoeas even though they are at their ideal weight (adding weight will make their apnoea worse, though).

It is important to remember that alcohol, or sedating or muscle-relaxing medications, can cause or contribute to OSA.

### Calculating Your BMI

Divide your weight in kilos by your height in metres squared. So if you weigh 53 kg and you are 1.6 metres in height, the formula is as follows:
$53 \div 1.6m^2 = 20.7$

| BMI | Weight Category |
| --- | --- |
| Less than 18.5 | Underweight |
| 18.5–24.9 | Normal weight |
| 25–29.9 | Overweight |
| 30 or greater | Obese |

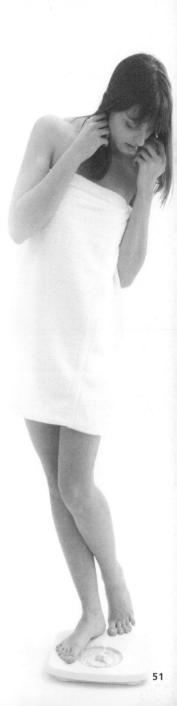

RIGHT *Persons with a high body mass index (BMI) are at greater risk of having obstructive sleep apnoea.*

## IS OSA BAD FOR ME?

Obstructive sleep apnoea is bad for you. There are very serious consequences of OSA, which stem from two main features of the disorder. First, after almost all apnoeas and many hypopnoeas there is a short arousal detected in EEG activity that results in a brief 2–3 second awakening. The majority of these are not recalled, but they wreak havoc on your sleep, which becomes fragmented as a result of these repeated interruptions. Since sleep-regulation machinery requires the brain to proceed through Stages 1 and 2 of sleep before arriving at slow-wave and REM sleep, persons with OSA have very reduced amounts of slow-wave sleep. The first period of REM sleep is delayed beyond the normal 90 minutes and overall REM time can be below normal as well. Interestingly, since the arousals are so brief, sleep duration can approach eight hours, but sleep quality is so diminished that people with OSA seldom feel as if they are getting a good night's sleep.

Second, the repeated drops in oxygen levels, rises in carbon-dioxide levels and changes in heart-rate rhythm are a strain on cardiac function. The combination of sleep fragmentation and cardiopulmonary strain may lead to hypertension, heart disease, stroke, mood and memory problems, headaches and daytime fatigue and sleepiness.

### POSSIBLE CONSEQUENCES OF OSA

About half of fatal car crashes are believed to be related to drivers nodding off; a large percentage of these are believed to be directly related to OSA. The risk of sudden cardiac death is greatly increased in habitual snorers and those who have OSA.

If you suspect that you may have OSA, go to a sleep specialist. The cost of a sleep evaluation, a diagnostic overnight sleep study and treatment for OSA is not inexpensive, but compared with a heart attack or car accident, the costs are reasonable.

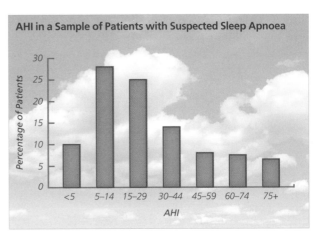

**AHI in a Sample of Patients with Suspected Sleep Apnoea**

*Percentage of Patients* (y-axis: 0, 5, 10, 15, 20, 25, 30)
*AHI* (x-axis: <5, 5–14, 15–29, 30–44, 45–59, 60–74, 75+)

ABOVE *Apnoea severity as defined by the apnoea-hypopnoea index (AHI) in a sample of 1,537 patients with suspected sleep apnoea. The AHI index corresponds to the number of apnoeas and hypopnoeas occurring per hour of sleep. (Unpublished data from Pigeon & Sateia.)*

## YOUR RISK OF HAVING OSA

The probability of having sleep apnoea increases with the number of risk factors you can identify. These include loud snoring, obesity, having a large neck size (17 inches or greater in men, or 16 inches or greater in women), being age 40 or older, having high blood pressure, smoking and alcohol use. In addition, if you have a family history of OSA or your ethnicity is African-American, Pacific-Islander, or Hispanic, these are considered risk factors. Other risk factors are if you wake up choking or gasping for air, a bed partner has observed pauses in your breathing while you sleep, or you experience general daytime sleepiness or fall asleep unintentionally during the day (as in watching television on the sofa at 3 p.m., for instance).

## DIAGNOSING OSA

The diagnosis of sleep apnoea can only be made by having an overnight sleep study. It is important to see a sleep specialist for a full sleep evaluation, which will include a thorough history of your sleep problems and an assessment of your overall health to determine what factors may be contributing to your sleep problems. In some cases, the sleep specialist may identify another medical condition or sleep disorder that may not require an overnight sleep study.

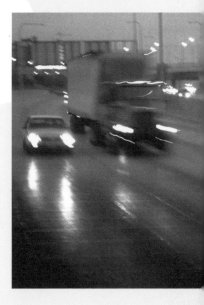

BELOW *The sleepiness that comes as a result of having sleep apnoea is associated with drowsy driving and motor vehicle accidents.*

An overnight sleep study enables the sleep specialist to determine whether obstructive sleep apnoea is present, and its severity. Following the sleep study, every apnoea, hypopnoea and arousal is scored. The number of apnoeas and hypopnoeas that occur are totalled and then divided by the number of hours of sleep that were achieved. The resulting number is called an apnoea-hypopnoea index (AHI). For example, if there are 80 events during eight hours of sleep, the AHI is ten. There are a number of standardized scoring rules and diagnostic criteria, but in general an AHI greater than or equal to five is considered to meet the diagnosis of OSA. OSA is divided roughly into mild, moderate and severe apnoea based on the level of the AHI. An AHI of 40 or greater is generally considered to be severe apnoea. In most sleep-disorder centres, which see thousands of patients per year, the average AHI is in the range of 25–30. This reflects that the average patient with OSA has 25–30 apnoeas or hypopnoeas per hour of sleep.

## TREATMENTS FOR OSA

Several of the available treatments for OSA are similar to those recommended for snoring. These include losing weight, positional therapy, oral appliances and surgery. They all tend to be more successful in curing OSA if the OSA is mild, though they can all decrease the severity of moderate or severe apnoea.

By far the most effective and widely used treatment for OSA is continuous positive airway pressure (CPAP) treatment. CPAP involves the delivery of filtered room air into the airway. It is delivered through a mask worn over the nose or face. The air gently blows into the back of the throat, preventing the airway from collapsing while you sleep. No collapse, no apnoeas or hypopnoeas. As a side benefit, any snoring usually resolves too.

A number of mask types are now available. You can choose the kind that provides the best fit and comfort for you. If the air in your home tends to be dry or your nasal and throat passages are dry following CPAP issue, a small heated humidifier can be added to the CPAP machine, and these are sometimes included as a standard feature. The CPAP unit itself is small enough to fit on a bedside table and sounds like a small bedroom fan. It also comes with a carry case so that it can be taken when travelling.

BELOW *Proper treatment of sleep apnoea can reverse its daytime consequences and restore energy and alertness.*

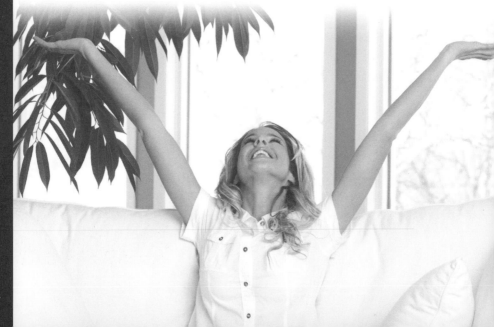

## Two Hypnograms of the Same Patient: One Before and One on the First Night of CPAP Use

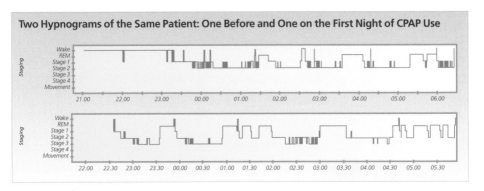

## A CPAP STUDY & LIFE WITH CPAP

The amount of air pressure needed to keep the airway open with CPAP is different for each person. The optimal pressure is arrived at during an overnight sleep study. If it is determined that a patient has sleep apnoea during the first half of the night, the sleep technicians will initiate CPAP during the second half of the night. Other times, if you have not slept enough to make a diagnosis or the severity of your apnoea is not clear until the latter part of the night, you will be asked to return for a CPAP study. In either case, the sleep technician carefully titrates the air pressure until the apnoeas and hypopnoeas dissipate. The sleep specialist then reviews the record and determines your optimal pressure.

## ADVANTAGES AND DISADVANTAGES OF CPAP

CPAP can have a dramatic effect on sleep quality. The number of arousals is reduced and sleep cycles become normal; slow-wave sleep may increase and REM sleep occurs at appropriate intervals. When CPAP is used every night, most patients feel better within 1–2 nights to 1–2 weeks. CPAP only cures OSA when it is used. Unless the underlying causes of OSA are addressed, OSA will recur every night. Some patients who were unsuccessful in prior weight-loss attempts find their improved sleep on CPAP provides the energy to lose enough weight to cure themselves of OSA. Although many patients swear by their CPAP, others swear about it, about inconvenience and discomfort. Rarely, people complain of claustrophobia when wearing the mask. Each individual must weigh the advantages and disadvantages of CPAP use in comparison with other treatment approaches.

ABOVE *Fragmented sleep, loss of Stage 3 and 4 sleep and delayed REM sleep (top panel) are reversed with CPAP therapy (bottom panel).*

### Tips for CPAP Use

• Seriously consider the risks of untreated sleep apnoea.
• List the benefits of improved sleep to your quality of life.
• Keep trying different masks until you have the right one for you.
• Ask your sleep specialist for heated humidification if dryness is a problem.
• Ask your sleep specialist if there is an apnoea support group in your area.
• If you develop a little claustrophobia, practise using the mask for brief periods, sitting up in a chair during the day, until the apprehension dissipates.

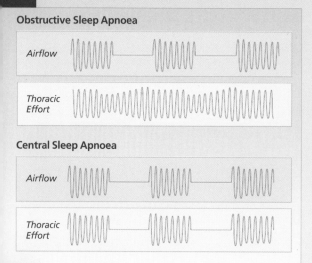

**Obstructive Sleep Apnoea**

*Airflow*

*Thoracic Effort*

**Central Sleep Apnoea**

*Airflow*

*Thoracic Effort*

ABOVE *While airflow ceases in both obstructive and central apnoeas, breathing effort continues during obstructive apnoeas, but ceases in central apnoeas.*

CENTRAL SLEEP APNOEA

Just as in OSA, central sleep apnoea (CSA) is marked by a cessation or limitation of breathing during sleep. The difference is that there is no obstruction of the airway involved in CSA. Instead, the airway remains open but breathing is interrupted. The 'central' in central sleep apnoea refers to the fact that the brain and the heart (which regulate breathing during sleep) are to blame for the pause in breathing.

As a result, the sights and sounds associated with CSA differ from OSA. Most importantly, while the airflow flatlines in a similar way, respiratory effort also flatlines in central apnoeas, whereas that effort reflected in abdominal and upper-chest movements continues during an obstructive apnoea. The end of a central apnoea is also gradual and quiet, as opposed to being sudden and accompanied by a gasp or snore. Other features are similar, such as a decrease in oxygen saturation, arousals at the end of apnoea and the presence of central hypopnoeas as well as central apnoeas. Snoring may also be present.

THE PREVALENCE OF CSA

The prevalence of CSA is far less common than OSA. Estimates from patients seen at sleep-disorder centres are that only 5–10 per cent of them have CSA, meaning that the overall prevalence in the general population is probably less than 1 per cent. Central sleep apnoea is quite rare in children and is mainly associated with older adults.

UNDERSTANDING CSA

Central sleep apnoea comes in a number of forms, some of which have their own unique causes. The unifying feature is that the regulation of breathing is malfunctioning, rather than the airway being obstructed. In primary CSA, the breathing pattern described above occurs repeatedly. The specific cause of the central dysregulation is not known, but it is rare and occurs in middle-aged or elderly men more than similarly aged women, with a tendency for being inherited. Some neurological conditions, such as Parkinson's disease, may cause primary CSA.

## VARIATIONS OF CSA

Cheyne-Stokes breathing pattern is a form of CSA defined by a rhythmic, choppy pattern of increases and decreases in breathing effort interspersed with central apnoeas. This occurs mainly in men over 60, especially in those with congestive heart failure or who have had a stroke. It is rarely seen in women and does not appear to be inherited.

Central sleep apnoea caused by medical conditions, but without the typical Cheyne-Stokes breathing pattern, may be due to a problem in the base of the brain where breathing is controlled. It can also be caused by heart and kidney problems, and much more rarely, by a variety of other medical conditions.

Drugs can cause CSA: they are almost exclusively opiates (pain medicines). The possibility of causing CSA increased after prolonged use. The breathing pattern can vary from complete apnoeas to cyclic increases and decreases, or elements of obstruction such as the breathing that is seen in OSA.

High-altitude periodic breathing is similar to the Cheyne-Stokes breathing pattern and, as the name implies, is caused directly by being at high altitudes. Some people sleeping at altitudes higher than about 4,500 metres (15,000 feet) will have this disorder. While most of us will have little reason to be at these heights, anyone sleeping above about 7,600 metres (25,000 feet) will be affected. Men are more prone to develop the condition because they seem to be more responsive to changes in the level of oxygen and carbon dioxide in their blood.

## TREATMENT FOR CSA

Treatments for CSA vary but positive airway pressure (PAP) delivered with CPAP (or its variant, Bi-PAP) is the most common treatment, although Adaptive Servo-Ventilation (ASV) is a recent and important advancement. Supplemental oxygen is sometimes used to treat some forms of central sleep apnoea, as is a change in medication if this is the primary cause of this sleep disturbance.

## OTHER BREATHING DISORDERS

There are a number of other sleep-related breathing disorders that warrant at least a brief overview. Most of these have a reduction in breathing during sleep and a related reduction in oxygen saturation, though the causes can vary.

### HYPOVENTILATION DISORDERS

A variety of disorders fall into the category of hypoventilation, or reduced breathing levels, during sleep. These may be due to lower-airway obstruction, which causes the lungs to work at less-than-full capacity. The single most common cause is cigarette smoking, which damages the lungs. Other contributors may be exposure to chemicals or pollutants. In addition, people with chronic bronchitis, emphysema, cystic fibrosis and other diseases affecting the lungs can develop hypoventilation.

Some people with neuromuscular and chest-wall disorders have difficulty breathing deeply. This results in higher levels of carbon dioxide in their blood, which they adapt to over time. Normally, people would breathe deeper and faster to get rid of the extra carbon dioxide, but people who have this sleep disorder are unable to do so.

One of the main concerns with hypoventilation disorders is the accompanying oxygen desaturation. Unlike in obstructive and central sleep apnoeas, there is little regular breathing during sleep, so that oxygen levels do not have time to recover. As a result, oxygen levels can remain at low levels for extended periods of time.

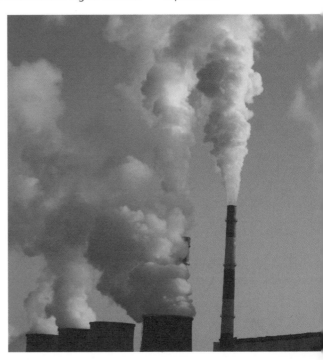

BELOW *Hypoventilation disorders may be caused by a number of factors, including exposure to pollutants.*

## TREATMENT OF HYPOVENTILATION DISORDERS

Treatment of hypoventilation disorders begins by treating the cause of the lower-airway obstruction, if one can be determined and treated. This will improve both daytime and night-time breathing patterns. Treatment choice also depends on determining not only the level of oxygen saturation, but also the level of carbon dioxide in the bloodstream.

Supplemental oxygen can be provided to help maintain oxygen levels. As there is the chance that adding extra oxygen may make carbon-dioxide levels worse, a sleep physician or pulmonologist must monitor the treatment closely. Oxygen may be delivered in conjunction with a CPAP or Bi-PAP device. Since hypoventilation may occur with sleep apnoea, this often happens.

## SLEEP PROBLEMS RELATED TO ASTHMA

Many people with asthma experience an exacerbation of their asthma at night. Visits to Accident and Emergency departments because of asthma tend to occur after midnight. Sleep for people with night-time asthma is very fragmented and of very poor quality. The few overnight sleep studies in people with night-time asthma show that they have more awakenings, shorter sleep durations and less deep sleep than normal sleepers.

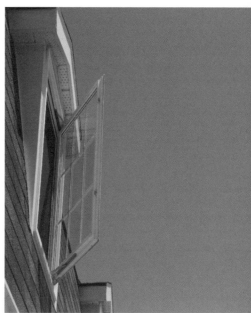

ABOVE *Asthma sufferers may improve both their sleep and their asthma symptoms by having a well-ventilated sleep environment.*

The primary contributor to night-time asthma appears to be related to the normal changes that occur in sleep, including a more relaxed (and thus smaller) airway, slightly increased inflammation of the airway, and more reactivity in the lungs to such things as allergens and pollutants. OSA can also be a cause of nocturnal asthma attacks.

## TREATMENT OF NOCTURNAL ASTHMA

Treatment of nocturnal asthma can begin with some preventive measures. These include enclosing mattresses and pillows in special covers, making sure the bedroom is properly ventilated and is not too dry, and minimizing exposure to allergens from pets, dust and so on. Some medications may also be helpful.

# SLEEP-RELATED MOVEMENT DISORDERS

There are several disorders of sleep that manifest as excessive movement during sleep. Many of us have the experience of tossing and turning during a poor night's sleep, but a sleep-related movement disorder is more pronounced and more regular. Movement disorders include restless leg syndrome, periodic limb-movement disorder, bruxism and a few less common disorders. All of these conditions can disrupt sleep to some degree.

## Causes of RLS

No precise cause of RLS has been determined. There does appear to be a genetic component to RLS, and a specific gene that accounts for about half of all cases for the disorder has been identified; but some people with the gene do not develop the disorder. Restless leg syndrome can also occur as a secondary feature of another medical condition. For instance, pregnancy, iron deficiency, kidney failure and some medications can cause or exacerbate RLS. It is also true that women have RLS at rates one and a half times to twice that of men.

## RESTLESS LEG SYNDROME

Restless leg syndrome (RLS) is a neurological condition that occurs in 5–10 per cent of the adult population and up to 2 per cent of children. Its primary feature is an overwhelming urge to move the legs during waking. It usually presents with an uncomfortable sensation in the legs, which is more pronounced during both periods of inactivity and the evening. In rare instances, the sensation may be present in other parts of the body. It is temporarily relieved by movement such as walking.

## SYMPTOMS & DIAGNOSIS OF RLS

The urge to move the legs is often associated with an uncomfortable feeling during periods of inactivity. This sensation has been described variably as tingling, itching, pulling, aching or a creepy-crawly feeling that is not relieved by scratching or touch. Symptoms may also include involuntary jerking of the limbs. This tends to become worse in the evening or at night. Both the sensation and the involuntary jerks are relieved by movement. Because these symptoms intensify at night, people with RLS tend to have difficulty falling or staying asleep. RLS is also associated with insomnia and therefore often produces chronic sleep loss, which leaves the sufferer with daytime feelings of fatigue, sleepiness or mild cognitive impairment. In addition, RLS is associated with another sleep movement disorder known as periodic limb-movement disorder, which is often (but not always) present during the sleep of those with RLS.

There is no specific test to identify RLS. Instead, your doctor or a sleep specialist will make the diagnosis based on your description of your symptoms. One test that is typically conducted, however, is a blood test to determine whether you might have an iron deficiency.

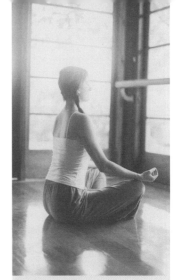

TREATMENTS OF RLS

Until recently there were no European Medicines Agency (EMEA)-approved drugs for the treatment of RLS, although some medications have been used for some time to treat the disorder. These medications fall into three main classes: opiate medications typically used to control pain, sedating medications used to improve sleep, and medications used to treat movement disorders such as Parkinson's disease, called dopaminergic agents. There are two drugs that act to increase dopamine in the system: ropinirole and mirapexin. These are typically prescribed in lower doses than when they are used for Parkinson's disease. Both drugs may cause side effects such as nausea and dizziness, and may cause patients to fall asleep with little, if any, warning, so precautions are necessary when taking them. In some patients, these drugs can eventually lead to a reappearance or worsening of RLS symptoms, which is known as augmentation.

In 1996, Drs Allen and Earley from Johns Hopkins University described the phenomenon called augmentation, in which RLS symptoms are more severe, spread to parts of the body other than the legs and begin earlier in the evening as a result of taking dopaminergic agents to treat RLS symptoms. If augmentation occurs, it can be managed with dose and medication adjustments.

**Tips for Managing Restless Leg Syndrome**

There are a number of self-directed activities for managing the symptoms of RLS, including walking, massaging the legs, stretching, hot or cold packs, vibration and acupressure. Relaxation techniques such as meditation or yoga have been known to alleviate symptoms. Also, treating an underlying cause, or effective pharmacological treatment of primary RLS and implementation of coping strategies, provide relief from most symptoms. However, sometimes medications need to be changed over time or the doses adjusted. Regular consultation with a physician is recommended.

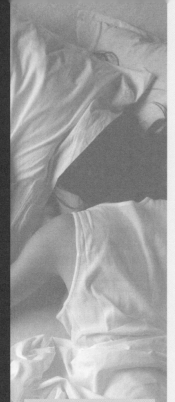

**Tips for Managing PLMs**

There are a few behavioural strategies that can help with PLMs. These include avoiding alcohol, caffeine and nicotine, which may contribute to RLS symptoms and/or PLMs; introducing a regular relaxation exercise into your daily routine; and engaging in daily, moderate levels of physical activity.

## PERIODIC LIMB-MOVEMENT DISORDER

Periodic limb-movement disorder (PLMD) is a condition in which repetitive movements of the legs and arms (though mostly in the legs) occur during sleep. However, some people can have periodic limb movements (PLMs) without having the full disorder, which requires the presence of a daytime or night-time consequence such as fatigue or sleepiness. The movements themselves are typically brief muscle twitches or small jerking movements with an upward flexing of the foot. They can occur approximately every 5–30 seconds, and often occur in clusters lasting anywhere from several minutes to several hours. PLMD is not especially common; approximately 1–4 per cent of adults are believed to have the disorder. Many patients with insomnia also experience a lot of tossing and turning.

### CAUSES OF PLMD

The precise cause of PLMD remains unknown, although specialists believe that there is some as-yet-undetermined underlying mechanism in the nervous system. As previously noted (see page 60), a significant number of individuals with RLS also have PLMs and PLMD. Occasionally PLMs may be an indicator of a serious medical condition, such as kidney disease, diabetes or anaemia. In children, attention-deficit hyperactivity disorder (ADHD) is associated with PLMs. By themselves, PLMs are not considered medically serious. They can, however, contribute to insomnia and/or to daytime fatigue or sleepiness when they cause awakenings during the night.

### SYMPTOMS & DIAGNOSIS OF PLMD

The main symptom of PLMD is, of course, the presence of PLMs during sleep. Unlike RLS, no discomfort in the limbs is necessary for the diagnosis of PLMD, although such discomfort may be present. Often sufferers are completely unaware of the night-time PLMs, and it is their bed partners' complaints that shed light on the problem. In addition to PLMs, a sleep complaint such as insomnia or daytime sleepiness must

LEFT *Many people have PLMs without experiencing the insomnia or daytime fatigue that is a feature of PLMD.*

be present for the diagnosis of PLMD. This diagnosis is made through a combination of patient (and bed partner) history, along with data from an overnight sleep study. Particularly astute bed partners may notice the movements are more likely to occur in the first half of the night, when non-REM sleep predominates. PLMs are much less common during REM sleep.

As is the case with sleep apnoea, there is a severity index for PLMs, which is calculated by counting the number of movements that occur per hour of sleep during an overnight sleep study. An index of greater than 15 movements per hour in adults, and greater than five in children, is generally considered the threshold for a diagnosis of PLMD. However, a greater number of movements is not related to greater levels of complaints by patients. By strict criteria, movements that are precipitated by respiratory disturbances (such as apnoea) should not be scored, and movements in this setting should not be considered periodic limb-movement disorder. Therefore, how the patient feels is as important in making the diagnosis and in considering treatment as the level of PLMs.

There is ongoing debate about whether disease severity, as assessed by the PLMs index, has any correlation with patient complaints. Again, in the absence of any patient complaints or the presence of any other sleep disturbance, the presence of PLMs does not require treatment.

## Treatments of PLMD

If there is an identified cause of the PLMD, such as RLS, then treatment of the primary condition is recommended. Several medications have been shown to be effective in treating PLMs, but treatment is only necessary when PLMs are accompanied by RLS, insomnia or daytime fatigue. The most recent guidelines consider the treatment for RLS and periodic limb movement of sleep to be the same. In the absence of limb discomfort, determining whether a medication is working can be somewhat challenging. Again, a bed partner's reports are critical, in addition to patient reports of any improvements in sleep and/or daytime sleepiness or fatigue.

There is some limited evidence that behavioural treatments for insomnia may also help in reducing PLMs. When a patient has insomnia, consideration of a medication for PLMD should be delayed until a course of insomnia treatment has been tried.

### Brief Arousals in EEG Brain Activity Associated with Leg Movements in a 30-Second Time Period

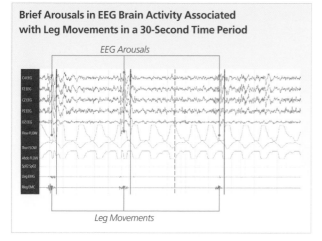

*EEG Arousals*

*Leg Movements*

LEFT *Leg movements, evidenced at the bottom of the graph, are immediately followed by brief EEG arousals lasting 1–3 seconds.*

# PRIMARY SLEEPINESS

Daytime sleepiness interferes with everyday life. Unintended lapses into drowsiness or sleep can be frustrating, embarrassing in social situations and lethal when driving.

### SYMPTOMS & DIAGNOSIS OF PRIMARY SLEEPINESS

Primary sleepiness is a chronic condition that must be present for at least three months and unrelated to a night-time sleep disorder. Daytime sleepiness is the critical symptom. Accurate diagnosis requires an overnight sleep study and a daytime sleep test in a laboratory. Results reveal whether there is a pathological level of sleepiness; an interview helps determine which disorder is present.

Narcolepsy occurs in less than 0.5 per cent of the population. It includes daytime sleepiness and evidence of REM sleep during daytime sleep tests. Individuals without narcolepsy seldom have REM sleep during daytime naps. One feature of narcolepsy is cataplexy – a sudden loss of muscle tone brought on by strong emotions, which lasts from a few seconds to a few minutes.

## Causes of Primary Sleepiness

Many sleep disorders cause daytime sleepiness, and thus these disorders can represent a major cause of sleepiness. Primary sleepiness, however, is not due to night-time sleep disorders. The additional causes of sleepiness essentially define the types of primary sleepiness disorders that exist, under a class of sleep disorders called 'hypersomnias of central origin'. These include narcolepsy, hypersomnia due to medical conditions or drugs, insufficient sleep syndrome, and idiopathic hypersomnias (code for 'we have no idea where this came from').

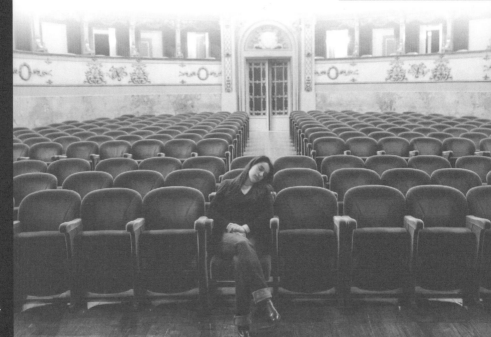

Additional features of narcolepsy can include sleep paralysis (temporary inability to move) upon waking, and dreamlike hallucinations prior to falling asleep and/or upon moving from sleep to wakefulness. Despite high levels of sleepiness, many patients with narcolepsy may also experience insomnia.

TREATMENTS OF PRIMARY SLEEPINESS

In rare cases when a medical condition or a drug is the culprit, sleepiness may be addressed by being better managed, by a change in medication, or treatment for substance abuse or withdrawal. Patients who are not giving themselves enough time to sleep only need to allow for more sleep opportunity.

Narcolepsy is not curable at this time, but the symptoms can be treated. Stimulants can help daytime alertness, and some anti-depressants can help with cataplexy, hallucinations and sleep paralysis. Any insomnia can be addressed. Brief naps in the day, a regular meal and exercise routine, avoiding alcohol and nicotine, and supportive counselling are helpful in treating your insomnia.

BOTTOM LEFT *Daytime dozing in public places, such as at the theatre or in meetings, could indicate an underlying sleep disorder.*

## Assessing Your Level of Daytime Sleepiness

How likely are you to doze off or fall asleep during the following situations, in contrast to just feeling tired? This refers to your usual way of life over the *past week*. Even if you have not done some of these things recently, figure out how they would have affected you. Use the following scale to choose the *most appropriate number* for each situation:

0 = would *never* doze
1 = *slight* chance of dozing
2 = *moderate* chance of dozing
3 = *high* chance of dozing

| Situation | Chance of Dozing |
|---|---|
| • Sitting and reading. | |
| • Watching TV. | |
| • Sitting, inactive in a public place (e.g. a theatre or a meeting). | |
| • As a passenger in a car for an hour without a break. | |
| • Lying down to rest in the afternoon, when circumstances permit. | |
| • Sitting and talking to someone. | |
| • Sitting quietly after a lunch without alcohol. | |
| • In a car, while stopped for a few minutes in traffic. | |

Total Score: _____ *

* A score of 10 or more indicates an above-average level of sleepiness

## CIRCADIAN-RHYTHM SLEEP DISORDERS

Optimal sleep occurs when one's desired sleep time matches the circadian rhythm of sleep and wakefulness. Sleep can be disrupted when the circadian timing system is altered, or when there is a mismatch between people's particular sleep–wake rhythms and the timing of social and environmental demands on them. As with the other classes of sleep disorders, there are several types of circadian-rhythm sleep disorders. We will address the four most common types.

SYMPTOMS & DIAGNOSIS OF CIRCADIAN DISORDERS
All circadian-rhythm sleep disorders have three symptoms in common that are required for a diagnosis. First, sleep is persistently or recurrently disturbed due specifically to an alteration in the sleep clock or to a mismatch between the internal sleep clock and the external social/occupational clock.

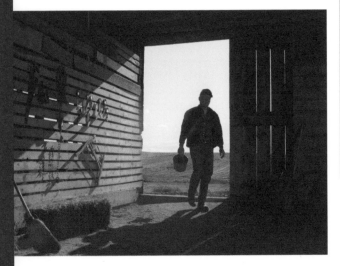

### Causes of Phase Advance

The precise causes of phase advance are not well detailed. However, it is believed that environmental factors may initiate the problem. For instance, someone with a very early work schedule (say a dairy farmer, or a school bus driver) may have had a normal sleep schedule that was altered because of work-schedule demands. Over time, their circadian rhythms were reset to this new work schedule. This is adaptive while they are working, but problematic if their work schedules change, and their circadian sleep rhythms remain fixed. Alternatively, exposure to either of the two main circadian shifters, light and melatonin, alter circadian rhythms. An ill-timed dose of melatonin, for instance, can phase advance an individual by 1–3 hours. There is also evidence that several circadian sleep disorders, including phase advance, are linked to a specific gene and can run in families.

LEFT *It may not be necessary to treat your phase advance if you can adapt your lifestyle to suit it.*

Second, the sleep disturbance leads to insomnia, excessive sleepiness or both. Third, the sleep disturbance leads to problems in one or more life areas. An overnight sleep study is not typically required to diagnose these disorders. Instead, data from self-reporting and from 2–3 weeks of daily reports of bedtime and rise time are sufficient. Additional information can describe and help determine the specific type of circadian-rhythm disorder.

## PHASE ADVANCE (TOO EARLY TO BED & TOO EARLY TO RISE)

The 'advance' in advanced sleep-phase disorder (or phase advance) refers to the sleep clock being set for sleep earlier than is normal. Persons with a phase advance have repeated difficulty staying awake until conventional bedtimes. For instance, they become sleepy in the late afternoon and have bed times of 6–9 p.m. They also become alert and are unable to remain asleep until conventional wake times (for example, they awake for the day at 4 a.m.). When allowed to sleep from, say, 8 p.m.–4 a.m., affected people typically achieve a normal amount of sleep (7.5–8 hours). When sleepiness is resisted and bedtime is delayed until later in the evening, however, the sleep clock still 'goes off' at 4 a.m. For a dairy farmer, this may seem like a perfect schedule, but it is less than ideal for most people. In addition, all other circadian rhythms related to sleep (the release of hormones and peaks and valleys of the body temperature curve) are also shifted earlier. Phase advance rarely occurs in children. It typically begins when someone is middle aged and is thought to affect about 1 per cent of adults.

## TREATMENTS OF PHASE ADVANCE

People who have adapted or can adapt their lifestyles to an early sleep schedule will not develop insomnia or sleepiness as a result of their phase advance. When lifestyle and schedule do not match, however, phase advance is usually addressed in one of several ways, each shifting the sleep clock to a more desirable schedule: by gradually and systematically delaying bedtime, taking melatonin in the morning, or using exposure to sunlight or bright light in the early evening. It is imperative that any of these approaches be appropriately timed, and that the dose of either melatonin or light intensity and its duration are tailored to the individual situation.

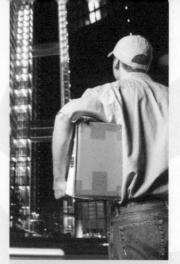

**Tips for Adapting to Phase Advance**

For those who wish to adapt better to a phase advance (as opposed to treating it), helpful and practical tips include:

• Considering the benefits of waking up early.

• Utilizing the early morning hours for one or more positive activities, such as relaxation, prayer or meditation, exercise or physical activity; preparing for the day, or catching up on reading or paperwork.

• Avoiding late-night activities.

• Avoiding late-afternoon or evening shifts at work.

• Refraining from consuming caffeine or stimulants in the late-afternoon or evening

• Avoiding using alcohol or drugs to stay asleep during the early morning hours.

## PHASE DELAY (THE NIGHT-OWL PROBLEM)

Delayed sleep-phase disorder (or phase delay) is the opposite of phase advance. In this circadian-rhythm disorder the typical sleep pattern is delayed by two or more hours, so that the sleep clock is shifted later at night and later in the morning. People with phase delay do not become sleepy at conventional sleep times for their age group. Their preferred sleep time may be something like 2–10 a.m. Thus, they are prototypical 'night owls'. When allowed to sleep on their preferred sleep schedules, individuals with phase delay are able to achieve their required amount of sleep. The telltale signs of phase delay include the inability to fall asleep at a standard time (for instance, 10 p.m.– midnight), coupled with difficulty getting up in the morning for standard school or work times. Unlike phase advance, phase delay typically develops in adolescence or early adulthood; approximately 10 per cent of young people have a phase delay.

Night owls can adjust to their phase delay if their work and/or social schedule permits. College students, for instance, can try to schedule only late-morning and afternoon classes, enabling them to study late into the night and to sleep late into the morning. When work, school and social schedules are not so accommodating, however, phase delay can lead to insomnia when sufferers try to get to sleep earlier than their sleep clocks will allow. They can also quickly develop daytime sleepiness from loss of sleep, having had to get up after less than their required amount of sleep.

### TREATMENTS OF PHASE DELAY

Like phase advance, phase delay can be treated by systematically changing the bedtime when lifestyle and schedule do not match (though with phase delay, the process is more trying). Bedtime is delayed by 2–3 hours per day for 5–7 consecutive days (so in the middle of this process the sleep period may be something like 3–11 p.m.). Once the desired bedtime is reached, the schedule is frozen and must be rigidly maintained. Exposure to natural or bright light shortly after waking up at the desired time in the morning is also helpful. Light exposure in the evening, on the other hand, should be avoided. It is best to receive advice from a sleep specialist to implement these strategies.

### Causes of Phase Delay

Again, specific mechanisms for phase delay are not well established. Voluntary changes from normal sleep schedules (staying up late and/ or sleeping in late) can lead to a mismatch between circadian drives and sleep drives, as well as promoting exposure to light at times of the day that can alter the sleep clock. A family pattern of phase delay is present in up to 40 per cent of people with phase delay, and a specific gene has been implicated in this disorder.

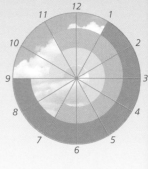

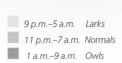

9 p.m.–5 a.m.  Larks
11 p.m.–7 a.m.  Normals
1 a.m.–9 a.m.  Owls

ABOVE *Preferred sleep times of 'night owls', normals and 'morning larks'.*

## Assessing Your Night-Owl or Morning-Lark Tendencies

Circle the most appropriate answer to each of the following questions.

**1** If you were able to plan your evening and had no commitments for the day after, at what time would you choose to go to bed?

| | |
|---|---|
| 8–9 p.m. | 5 |
| 9–10.15 p.m. | 4 |
| 10.15 p.m.–12.30 a.m. | 3 |
| 12.30 a.m.–1.45 a.m. | 2 |
| 1.45 a.m.–3.00 a.m. | 1 |

**2** If you have gone to bed several hours later than normal, but don't have to get up early the following day, which is the most likely outcome?

| | |
|---|---|
| You will wake up at the usual time and not fall asleep again | 4 |
| You will wake up at the usual time and doze thereafter | 3 |
| You will wake up at the usual time, but will fall asleep again | 2 |
| You will not wake up until later than usual | 1 |

**3** You have a two-hour test to take, which will be mentally exhausting. If you were free to choose, at what time would you take the test?

| | |
|---|---|
| 8–10 a.m. | 4 |
| 11 a.m.–1 p.m. | 3 |
| 3–5 p.m. | 2 |
| 7–9 p.m. | 1 |

**4** A friend has asked you to join him twice a week for a gym workout at 10–11 p.m. Bearing in mind only how you normally feel in the evening, how would you perform?

| | |
|---|---|
| Very well | 1 |
| Reasonably well | 2 |
| Poorly | 3 |
| Very poorly | 4 |

**5** One hears about 'morning' and 'evening' types of people. Which of these types do you consider yourself to be?

| | |
|---|---|
| Definitely morning type | 4 |
| More a morning than an evening type | 3 |
| More an evening than a morning type | 2 |
| Definitely an evening type | 1 |

### Morning or Evening Person?

Sum your answers and determine what range of morning–evening *chronotype* you are closest to:

| 5 | 21 |
|---|---|
| 'Night-owl' tendency | 'Morning-lark' tendency |

(Adapted from: 'A Self Assessment Questionnaire to Determine Morningness–Eveningness in Human Circadian Rhythms' by J.A. Horne and O. Ostberg, *International Journal of Chronobiology*, 1976, Vol. 4, 9–110)

## Flying Across Multiple Time Zones

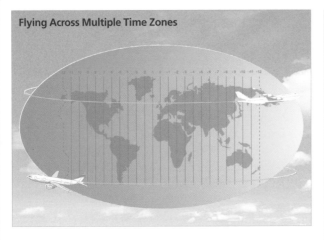

## JET LAG

Jet lag is a circadian-rhythm sleep disorder that occurs when you travel to somewhere that is several time zones removed from where your air travel originated. It is a mismatch between your sleep clock and the actual time clock of your destination. Owing to the speed of travel, the sleep clock does not have time to adjust right away to the new time. Jet lag is a temporary condition that appears 1–2 days after air travel across at least two time zones. Its severity and duration depend on the number of time zones crossed and the direction of travel. Flying east tends to be harder to adjust to than flying west. Jet lag can also be exacerbated by loss of sleep due to the travelling, air pressure and quality, prolonged uncomfortable seating positions, stress, and excessive caffeine or alcohol.

The effects of jet lag are well known to even the infrequent traveller and include the following: disturbed sleep at night, diminished alertness and increased sleepiness during the day, difficulty in functioning normally during the day, mild illness or cold-like symptoms, nausea and/or stomach problems and menstrual symptoms in women who travel often.

ABOVE *Jet lag is worse when flying east. It can take approximately one day per time zone for the body clock to adjust.*

## Recovery from Jet Lag

It generally takes about one day per time zone for your body clock to fully adjust to the local time. Crossing more than six time zones can require even more time for your body to adapt, especially if the sleep clock shifts in the opposite direction from the direction of travel. Exposure to light at inappropriate times for optimal recovery from jet lag can also affect the time it takes to get used to the new time zone.

Although no one is spared some level of jet lag, some people are able to adjust more quickly than others to rapid shifts in time zones. Older adults tend to have more difficulty with jet lag. Frequent travellers, such as pilots, flight attendants, business travellers and professional athletes, are subject to repeated bouts of jet lag, which can complicate recovery. Some professional, Olympic and university sports teams have recognized jet lag's effect on performance and, where possible within the parameters of their schedules, have adjusted travel times and even practice times to optimize the conditions for maximal alertness and performance on the day/night of their events.

## CAN I DO ANYTHING ABOUT JET LAG?

Jet lag can be minimized to some extent by addressing controllable factors before, during and after travel across time zones. If optimal functioning is desired for a certain event on a certain day (and scheduling permits), arriving two or more days ahead of time is an effective strategy. If this is not possible, the time of the event should be scheduled to coincide with times when you will be most alert on your first day at your destination. In other words, schedule according to your 'home' time, because your sleep clock will not have adjusted on the first day of travel.

Another useful strategy to employ is to begin to slightly adjust both your sleep and meal times towards the time in your destination several days before you travel. For instance, for a flight from Britain to the United States, the traveller can begin delaying meal and bedtimes by 30–60 minutes per day for 3–4 days. This will not completely make up the time difference, but it can begin to adjust the sleep clock to the destination time prior to departure. It is also possible to use melatonin or light exposure to assist this process, which should be done under the advice of a sleep specialist for optimal timing and dosing (and to avoid unintended shifts in the sleep clock).

Drink fluids to prevent dehydration, and avoid alcohol and caffeine. Depending on the length of the flight, pack a healthy meal or snack to supplement airline food if necessary.

## CAN SLEEPING DURING THE FLIGHT HELP?

Napping on the flight can be challenging, for two main reasons. First, because sleeping on an aeroplane is never a sure bet. Second, because even if sleep is possible, whether it will be helpful depends on whether the sleep clock has begun to shift before departure, on the time and duration of the flight, and on the time of arrival relative to the sleep clock. In general, sleeping on the plane should be avoided if it occurs less than 4–6 hours prior to your intended bedtime at your destination. Otherwise, a 20–40-minute nap may be quite helpful. A guideline for a longer sleep period on the plane is impossible without considering all the specific timing factors of your travel. If some amount of sleep is desired or planned during the flight, the savvy traveller will come prepared with helpful items, such as earplugs and eyeshades.

**Tips for Coping with Jet Lag**

Upon arrival, match your sleep schedule immediately to the local time. If your bedtime is 11 p.m. and you are travelling westward, staying up until 11 p.m. local time may be difficult because your home time is later. Exposure to daylight and modest physical activity will help (avoid using caffeine to help you stay up).

If travelling eastward, the local time may again be 11 p.m., but you may not be sleepy for hours. Options here include going to bed when sleepy, but set the alarm for the local wake-up time that you wish to be on, or take a sleep medication (for 1–2 nights) to help you fall asleep an hour or two before you would otherwise be sleepy.

These methods work best when traveling over a few time zones. Travelling over six or more time zones needs more attention to the details of the travel. If in doubt, consult a sleep specialist.

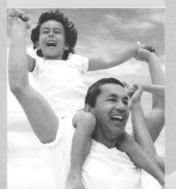

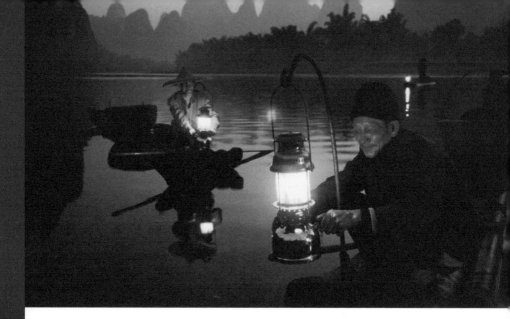

ABOVE *Shift work increased dramatically with the industrial revolution, but also has a long history in more traditional occupations such as fishing.*

## SLEEP PROBLEMS RELATED TO SHIFT WORK

Sailors, herdsmen and soldiers have worked nights for centuries, but the dawn of modern shift work began in 1879 when Thomas Edison invented the electric light bulb. Shift-work sleep disorder is a circadian-rhythm sleep disorder caused by a work schedule that occurs in the normal sleep period. Working when your sleep clock is ready for sleep, and trying to sleep when your sleep clock is not expecting it, creates a mismatch. A shift-work sleep disorder is diagnosed when insomnia and/or sleepiness arises from the mismatch, when it persists for at least a month and when it causes problems with work or social functioning.

Several tests have been conducted in sleep laboratories in which participants were not permitted to determine the time from clocks, sunlight or any other time cues. In these studies, participants slept approximately two hours less during daytime hours, despite being awake for an extended period, than when they were allowed to sleep during their normal sleep times. This showed that it is nearly impossible to attain the required amount of sleep when the sleep clock has not adjusted to a shift-work schedule. The problems are more pronounced among workers on the evening or late shifts (as opposed to late afternoon to evening shifts).

The problem is less pronounced when shift workers do successfully shift their sleep clock to match their work schedule. However, most revert to normal sleep schedules on their days off, essentially reshifting their clocks. Also, exposure to sunlight can quickly shift the sleep clock back to a normal day-night rhythm. Insufficient sleep for 3–5 days in a row quickly creates sleepiness.

## THE IMPACT OF SHIFT-WORK SLEEP DISORDER

Sleep problems can exacerbate other problems related to shift work, such as stomach and digestive problems, mood and memory problems, and hypertension and heart disease. Social functioning can also be affected. The non-shift-working spouse is often at home alone at night, and if the children are in school the only time when the shift-working parent may see them is when they are trying to sleep. Spouse and parent roles are disrupted if the work occurs on weekends. Planning social events is difficult due to work and sleep schedules, and the shift worker may also suffer isolation from day-working friends and community organizations, which assume that evenings and weekends will be free for meetings. When sleep is disturbed, shift workers have little energy to engage in social activities anyway. They have reduced alertness because of sleepiness from disturbed sleep and the havoc created on their sleep clock, and tend to have higher rates of work- and motor-vehicle-related accidents than their day-shift counterparts. Also, using drugs or alcohol to improve sleep can lead to substance abuse.

### Tips for Managing Shift Work

If the shift work is long-term, employers can reduce the number of times workers change shifts, change shifts forward in time instead of back when workers rotate through schedules, give regular rest periods, offer exercise breaks, make nutritious food available and use bright lighting in work areas. Workers can avoid high-carbohydrate foods when at work, make judicious use of caffeine and wear full sunlight-blocking glasses for the trip home. Sleep periods should begin directly on arriving home. For some, a large sleep period right away and then a nap later in the day increases their total sleep time over a 24-hour period. No one should interfere with their sleep periods. The bedroom should be totally dark, and earplugs and/or a sound machine can protect sleep. If insomnia at home or sleepiness at work persist, explore medication or behavioural strategies with a sleep specialist.

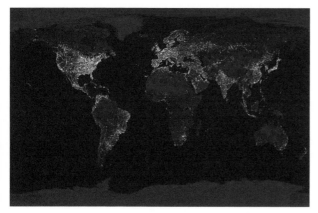

LEFT *A compilation of night-time satellite images. Even non-shift workers can be exposed to light sources 24 hours a day. Prolonged exposure to such lighting at night can contribute to shifts in our biological clock.*

# PARASOMNIAS

The parasomnias consist of a group of sleep disorders with the defining feature of an undesired physical event or experience that occurs during some phase of sleep. Some of these events can be quite benign, whereas others can result in injury, disrupted sleep and undesired social consequences – and can seriously scare parents when they present in a child. All the events begin with the central nervous system being activated. This activation is transmitted into the autonomic nervous system, which controls things below our level of consciousness (including some muscle activity), and can result in very complex behaviours. Although the behaviours may sound and look like conscious acts, there is no deliberate conscious control.

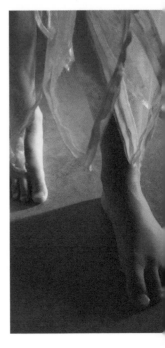

ABOVE *Parasomnias occur during the deep stages of sleep, and the sleeper is unaware of these nocturnal activities.*

## SLEEP TALKING

Sleep talking (or somniloquy) occurs when you talk out loud during sleep. The subject matter can vary widely and tends to be harmless or to make little sense, although it may sometimes be offensive. The talking can also occur repeatedly and/or be quite loud, which can disrupt the sleep of a bed partner or room-mate. At other times it may be barely audible.

Sleep talking is very common and mostly harmless. It occurs in about 50 per cent of young children and 5 per cent of adults, with no difference between the rates in males and females. It appears to run in families. People who only begin sleep talking as adults may sometimes have another sleep disorder, a medical condition, be on new medication or abusing a drug, have a mental health condition or be under a new or increased level of stress. On its own, sleep talking seldom requires treatment.

### When Sleep Talking Occurs

Sleep talking can occur by itself or in the context of another parasomnia, in which case it is typically much more dramatic and is loud, emotional, and/or profane. Sleep talking may occur in any stage of non-REM or REM sleep. Surprisingly, it is still not known whether or not it is closely linked to dreaming.

## SLEEPWALKING

Sleepwalking (or somnambulism) occurs when you get up from bed and walk around while still asleep. It can also involve a series of complex actions. Before walking, some people may sit up in bed and look around in a confused manner, while others may immediately jump up from bed. The eyes are usually open, but have a 'not all there' look to them. Actions vary from those that make little sense, such as moving an object to an odd place, to those that are part of a daily routine, such as doing the dishes or preparing (and eating) a snack. Behaviour may also turn hostile or violent. In rare cases, a child may walk to a neighbour's house, or an adult may get in a car and drive away.

A sleepwalker may return to bed while still asleep, having never woken up or realized what has happened. The event can also end suddenly, leaving the person somewhat confused and potentially in an awkward place or situation.

Sleepwalking occurs in non-REM sleep, rarely or frequently, often in the first third of sleep when slow-wave sleep predominates. It occurs in 15 per cent of children and 4 per cent of adults, with no gender differences. In children, sleepwalking is seen as fairly normal. Rates peak by the age of 8–12 years. There is a strong genetic/family link to sleepwalking: rates double if one parent was a sleepwalker. The main risk from sleepwalking is injury to self, a bed partner or others in the home. Children may walk to an open window or balcony, or go outside in bad weather. A person may leave the cooker on. In adults, men are more likely to be aggressive when they sleepwalk. The sleepwalker can also disrupt the sleep of parents, room-mates or the bed partner.

## ASSESSING AND DEALING WITH SLEEPWALKING

Consultation with a specialist is needed for children or adults who engage in complex and dangerous sleepwalking behaviours. A thorough review of possible causes of sleepwalking is necessary, including other sleep disorders, medical conditions, and life circumstances. Assessment may include a videotaped overnight sleep study to help determine the nature of the parasomnia.

Give sleepwalkers plenty of space and call their names gently to wake them if they appear to be putting themselves at risk for injury. Since most children typically 'grow out of it', parents may simply need to take precautions to avoid the possibility of injury.

### Parental Tips for Keeping a Sleepwalking Child Safe

• Tie a bell to your child's bedroom door to alert you when the door is opened.
• Calmly help your child return to bed during a sleepwalking episode.
• Install safety gates at the top of any stairs, and lock all windows in the house.
• Install locks out of your child's reach on all basement or external doors.
• If episodes regularly occur at the same time of night, briefly wake your child just before that time.

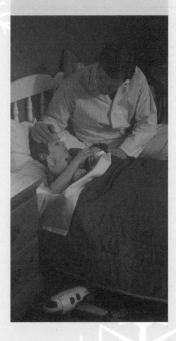

## SLEEP TERRORS

Sleep terrors are also called night terrors and are an extreme fear response that may include screaming and shouting, kicking and punching, and attempts to protect oneself from a perceived threat. Children tend to stay in their bed or bedroom, whereas adults may attempt to run away and/or engage in violent acts. In the midst of a sleep terror, a person's eyes are open and intense-looking, the heart is racing and the breathing is heavy. The person is difficult to wake up, and awakes confused, with little or no memory of the event. As with sleepwalking, sleep terrors occur during non-REM sleep and typically during the first third of the night. In adults, sleep terrors can also occur during REM sleep, and the person may have partial recall of a frightening dream.

Although less common than sleepwalking, sleep terrors are considered normal and occur in around 6–7 per cent of children and in 2 per cent of adults. There is a strong genetic/family link. Children with sleep terrors also often sleep talk and sleepwalk. Many adults with sleep terrors have a history of mood or anxiety disorders. Sleep terrors can occur because of another sleep disorder that fragments sleep, or when someone is sleep-deprived.

Sleep terrors in children generally do not require treatment, but parents should pay attention to safety. Children may be embarrassed by their sleep terrors, which can greatly affect their relationships with others (imagine, for instance, having a sleep-terror episode when away at camp or starting university). In addition, serious injury can occur while trying to flee from bed or to fight, particularly in adults. For these reasons, sleep terrors in adults should be evaluated by a sleep specialist.

## CONFUSIONAL AROUSALS

Confusional arousals occur when someone exhibits confusing behaviour on waking, such as slow speech, confused thinking, poor memory and flat responses to questions. There is no memory of the episode afterwards. Episodes in children may seem bizarre and frightening to parents. Children can look confused, appear dazed and may become agitated by attempts to comfort them. Most episodes last only 5–15 minutes, but can last up to 30–40 minutes in some youths. In adults, they may last for a few minutes or a few hours. In rare cases they may include very inappropriate, hostile or aggressive behaviour.

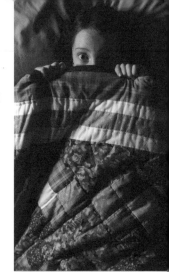

**Parental Tips for Managing a Child's Sleep Terrors**

• Remember that, distraught as your child appears, he or she will not recall the event and is safe.
• Do not attempt to wake your child.
• Remain calm to avoid frightening your child when he or she does wake up.
• Watch your child to make sure he or she remains safe.
• Wait near your child until he or she returns to normal sleep.
• If episodes occur regularly at the same time of night, briefly wake your child just before that time.

ABOVE *Sleep terrors are very frightening for parents to observe, but the main concern is to keep the sleeper safe.*

Confusional arousals tend to occur as you wake directly from slow-wave sleep during some portion of the night, but can also occur while waking in the morning. They are present in about 15 per cent of children (though less common after the age of five) and in 3–4 per cent of adults (and less common after the age of 35). The specific mechanism of the disorder is unknown, but family history plays a role. Several causes include being forced awake, sleep deprivation, various sleep disorders, shift work, stress or worry, alcohol or drug abuse, or bipolar disorder.

Confusional arousals are fairly harmless in children, but can cause significant stress and personal problems in the home and may sometimes be dangerous in teens and adults. Morning confusional arousals can cause school or work absenteeism and make for a less than fully alert driver. Treatment should be sought in adult cases, beginning with a thorough review of possible causes and a videotaped overnight sleep study. Treating other sleep disorders and addressing other potential causes is the next step, followed by introducing one of the anti-depressant or sleep medications that are proven to be helpful.

REM SLEEP BEHAVIOUR DISORDER

REM sleep behaviour disorder (RBD) is the acting out – often dramatically and/or violently – of vivid dreams during REM sleep. RBD may be confused with sleepwalking or sleep terrors, but tends to occur during the last half of the night. It arises only from REM sleep and the sleeper is easily awakened. On waking, the person has good memory of the dream, which is literally being acted out in some way. Episodes tend to become worse over time and eventually lead to injury to the sleeper or bed partner.

**About RBD**

REM sleep behaviour disorder can occur at any age, but mostly develops after the age of 50 and is present in less than 1 per cent of adults. Causes include sleep deprivation, anything else that increases the intensity or amount of REM sleep, severe stress and some neurological disorders such as Parkinson's disease. REM sleep behaviour disorder can only be diagnosed from an overnight sleep study. It tends to respond to sedating medications, though taking safety precautions in the home to avoid serious injury is highly recommended.

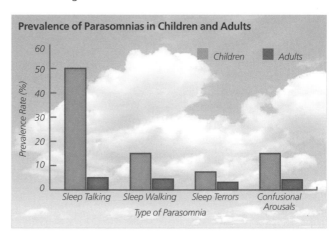

**Prevalence of Parasomnias in Children and Adults**

# NIGHTMARES

Nightmares are disturbing, visual dreams that occur during sleep (almost exclusively in REM sleep) and usually wake the dreamer. The content of nightmares varies, but they often involve themes of great threat, danger or loss to the dreamer, or witnessing something horrific or frightening. Almost everyone has had one or more nightmares at some time, but a nightmare disorder develops when nightmares occur frequently and cause some distress. Having frequent nightmares can cause someone to fear or avoid going to sleep, worry about having a nightmare, have difficulty in initiating sleep, or in returning to sleep after a nightmare. Sleep loss can lead to daytime sleepiness and a higher probability of nightmares the next night.

Nightmares are fairly common in young children; their frequency reaches a peak by about ten years of age and then decreases steadily. At least half of adults report an occasional nightmare, which lessens in both frequency and intensity as they grow older. Nightmare disorder, however, occurs in only 2–8 per cent of adults.

## CAUSES OF FREQUENT NIGHTMARES

Frequent nightmares in adults – as opposed to the fairly normal occurrence of the occasional nightmare – are often associated with a mental health condition. The most common of these is post-traumatic stress disorder (PTSD) stemming from a traumatic event. Nightmares that replicate the trauma or bear some semblance to it are a very common feature of acute reactions to a trauma and chronic PTSD. Again, the difference between someone experiencing a few disturbing dreams or nightmares following a severe car accident, and someone in the same vehicle experiencing repetitive and trauma-replicating dreams, is quite profound. The former may be having a normal reaction to a traumatic event, with the disturbing dream or nightmare being an attempt to regulate emotion and make sense of the trauma, whereas the latter is a failure of that process.

Other causes of frequent nightmares include some sleep disorders and some medications. Increased stress has also been directly associated with an increase in nightmares.

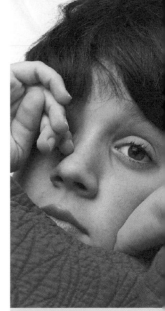

## Parental Tips for Managing a Child's Nightmares

• Install a nightlight in your child's room.
• Let your child sleep with a special blanket or soft toy.
• Comfort your child when he or she wakes from a nightmare.
• Let your child know that nightmares are normal, and talk about the content of the dreams/nightmares with him or her.

ABOVE *Nightmares are so common among children that they are considered a normal experience. They tend to decrease in frequency as the child gets older.*

## TREATING NIGHTMARES

When a nightmare disorder is related to another sleep disorder, medications, trauma or PTSD, it is important that these conditions receive attention because their treatment may alleviate nightmares. When PTSD is treated, for instance, nightmares dissipate in nearly three-quarters of patients. Regardless of the cause of the nightmares, all people with nightmare disorder need to manage stress in their lives and attempt to obtain regular adequate sleep.

### TARGETED TREATMENTS FOR NIGHTMARES

Targeted treatments for nightmares include mediations and some form of counselling or psychotherapy. In particular, there are two promising approaches to treating frequent trauma-related nightmares that deserve further discussion. The first is an old medication used traditionally as blood-pressure medicine called Prazosin, which greatly reduces the severity of nightmares and is safe and non-habit-forming. You will not see Prazosin advertised, because the patent on the drug expired and it is now available in generic form and is very inexpensive. The only downside of Prazosin is that it is not curative; when it is discontinued, the nightmares tend to return.

The second promising treatment is a set of therapy techniques that fall under the heading of 'Imagery Rehearsal Therapy'. There are several variants of this approach, but in all cases the dreamers are instructed to write down one of their nightmares and rehearse it by reading or imagining it during the daytime. Sometimes the patient is instructed to rewrite some aspect of the dream narrative and to rehearse it during the day. When one or more of these techniques is used, the nightmare can be cured. In other words, the reduction in frequency and intensity of the nightmares is maintained, even after the treatment has ended.

### Helpful Tips to Manage (or Avoid) All Parasomnias

• If you have an untreated (or poorly treated) sleep disorder, medical condition, anxiety, depression or heavy stress, get it treated!

• While at your doctor's surgery, review all medications that you are currently taking to determine whether any of them might cause or contribute to a parasomnia. If one of your medications happens to be a sleeping pill, make sure you are using it according to the prescription (and especially do not combine it with alcohol).

• Abide by what should be considered part of any health-care reform: don't drink alcohol (or at least severely limit your intake), just say 'no' to drugs, and get a full night of sleep every night (in other words, don't get sleep-deprived).

• If your work schedule causes poor sleep (for example, shift work) or you are regularly forced awake by pagers, scanners or phone calls about work, consider what changes might be made to better protect your sleep.

Insomnia is the most common sleep disorder. It is well defined and many of its features are experienced by nearly all insomnia sufferers. Yet, there is also tremendous variation in how insomnia presents and in individual experiences of insomnia. In this chapter, we undertake the task of determining whether your sleep problems are indeed related to insomnia. Equally important, we will explore the several types of insomnia that exist and determine what type of insomnia may be active in your case, as well as the particular subtype that you may be experiencing. This process of identification and categorizing will aid you in choosing and constructing the appropriate treatment programme for your situation.

# CHAPTER 3
# WHAT IS INSOMNIA?

# WHAT IS INSOMNIA?

Insomnia is a sleep disorder marked primarily by difficulty in initiating and/or maintaining sleep. Its development can be somewhat complex (or at least involve multiple factors). This is because of the many inputs into the sleep system that can become dysregulated, and to the variety of individual behaviours and thought practices that interact with the biological inputs to sleep. The assessment of insomnia involves a thorough review of how the factors that are required for normal sleep can become dysregulated. Although insomnia has several core features, there are various types of insomnia and even subtypes, which are important to identify to develop and personalize treatment.

**Daytime Impairments & Symptoms Associated with Insomnia**

- Low energy or fatigue.
- Lack of motivation.
- Attention, concentration or memory problems.
- Poor performance in school, work or social endeavours.
- Mood disturbance or irritability.
- Daytime sleepiness.
- Susceptibility to making errors at work.
- Having accidents at work, home or while driving.
- Tension, headaches or stomach aches.
- Frustration, worry or concerns about sleep.

## DEFINITIONS & SYMPTOMS OF INSOMNIA

Insomnia is a common problem. Almost everyone experiences a few nights of insomnia once in a while. Up to 30 per cent of adults have some symptoms of insomnia, and one-third of these (about 10 per cent of the population) have persistent insomnia.

A sleep disturbance is defined as insomnia when a person meets three requirements: first, difficulty falling asleep, difficulty staying asleep, waking up too early, and/or having poor-quality sleep; second, these problems occur despite adequate opportunity and circumstances for sleep; and third, there is some form of daytime impairment because of the sleep problem. An overnight sleep study is not required to make a diagnosis of insomnia.

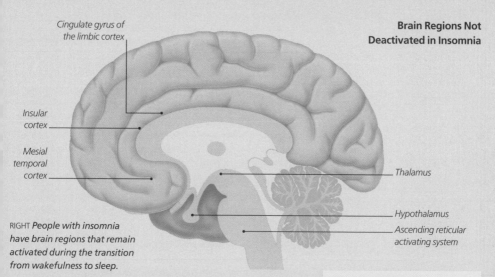

Cingulate gyrus of
the limbic cortex

Insular
cortex

Mesial
temporal
cortex

Thalamus

Hypothalamus

Ascending reticular
activating system

RIGHT *People with insomnia
have brain regions that remain
activated during the transition
from wakefulness to sleep.*

## CAUSES OF INSOMNIA

Insomnia can have many causes. The most common is stress
due to a new life event. Around 50–80 per cent of patients with
a chronic pain condition such as low back pain, arthritis or
fibromyalgia develop insomnia. High rates of insomnia also follow
difficult medical procedures such as chemotherapy and heart
surgery, and in conditions such as diabetes, multiple sclerosis,
asthma, and some sleep disorders, including sleep apnoea and
restless leg syndrome. It occurs in psychological conditions such
as depression, bipolar disorder, anxiety disorders and PTSD (see
page 78). Drug and alcohol dependence and the initial stages of
recovery can cause it, and it can be a side effect of medications.

Some biological mechanisms are believed to cause insomnia
when they are not working normally, including two mechanisms
central to proper sleep regulation. First, a disturbance in the sleep
clock – whether or not it is severe enough to be called a circadian-
rhythm disorder – can cause insomnia. This occurs when there is
a mismatch between the desired sleep time and when the sleep
clock is 'allowing' sleep to occur. Fighting the altered sleep clock
leads to an inability to initiate or maintain sleep. Second, if the
sleep homeostat (see page 22) is not properly set, a person may
not become tired enough to fall asleep, and/or may wake up
after a few hours and be too alert to fall back to sleep.

### The Arousal System

Many people with insomnia
have elevated levels of arousal,
particularly when they are
trying to go to sleep, including
raised levels of stress hormones
at sleep onset, and overactive
brain regions that are not
shutting down. Thinking styles
and behaviours may also cause
insomnia. Worriers, or people
who think a lot, often develop
insomnia when they take
thoughts and worries to bed.
People may also engage in
activities that set the stage
for insomnia when they keep
erratic sleep schedules or stay
in bed when they are awake
for excessive lengths of time.
Any or all of the listed causes
may interact in ways that lead
to new or worsening insomnia.

## TYPES OF INSOMNIA

Insomnia can vary: it may be acute or chronic, it may stand alone or it may be related to another condition. It may also have some specific features.

### ACUTE & CHRONIC INSOMNIA

Acute insomnia (also known as short-term insomnia or adjustment insomnia) occurs in response to an identifiable stressor and typically lasts for 1–3 months. This insomnia tends to resolve once the stressor has passed or the individual has adapted to it. Insomnia that lasts for a few days is not something to be concerned about and should be viewed as normal. When insomnia lasts for anywhere from several weeks to one or two months, there is reason for concern that the acute insomnia may develop into a chronic condition.

Chronic insomnia lasts for three months or more. It is concerning because once it becomes chronic, insomnia does not typically resolve on its own. For instance, in one study, the average chronicity of the disorder in a group of research subjects was ten years. What is more, when they were assessed five years later, 88 per cent continued to report insomnia. Insomnia, then, is a condition that needs to be addressed before it becomes chronic.

### PRIMARY & 'COMORBID' INSOMNIA

Insomnia may also present on its own, which we call 'primary' insomnia, or may be caused or worsened by another condition, which we call 'comorbid' insomnia. The number of possible comorbid insomnia types is large, so it is estimated that primary insomnia represents only about 10–20 per cent of all insomnias. The nature of the co-occurring condition can modify the features of insomnia.

### EXAMPLES OF UNIQUE FORMS OF COMORBID INSOMNIA

Although many forms of comorbid insomnia respond well to treatments that are used for primary insomnia, these treatments

**Precipitants of Chronic Insomnia**

Psychiatric 43%
Primary 22%
Movement Disorder 6%
Circadian 11%
Breathing 6%
Substance Disorder 6%
Other 6%

ABOVE *Primary insomnia consists of one-fifth of all insomnia complaints, while the rest are associated with another condition.*

RIGHT *Stressful life events, even happy ones such as a wedding, may be the initial cause of an acute episode of insomnia.*

work even better when they are adjusted to fit the specific kind of comorbid insomnia in question. This is because the comorbid disorders themselves can complicate insomnia in unique ways.

Chronic pain conditions can create a vicious pain–sleep cycle in which poor sleep causes increased pain sensitivity and increased pain causes poor sleep. Patients with chronic pain often have difficulty finding a comfortable position to sleep in, or may wake up stiff and sore when they do sleep well. Their chronic pain condition may make them less physically active, which can affect sleep. They may also gain weight and develop sleep apnoea. Pain medications can also have sleep consequences. Living with pain, and the ways it can alter one's life, is a stressor that does not go away if the pain persists. We have seen that stress has a very prominent role to play in disrupting sleep. It would make sense, then, to pay attention to the factors that are specific to chronic pain when we define and set out to treat insomnia in someone with a chronic pain condition.

A sleep research laboratory in Rochester, New York, showed that addressing these specific factors as part of an insomnia treatment resulted in superior benefits to chronic-pain patients on their ratings of sleep, pain and mood than treating only the insomnia or only the pain. This makes sense, of course, but with one-size-fits-all mentalities such commonsense approaches can sometimes be lost.

### Psychological Comorbidity

One example of psychological comorbidity from insomnia is related to trauma or PTSD (see page 78). Insomnia is present in 80 per cent or more of patients with PTSD and has unique features not normally seen with other insomnia types . The first is nightmares, which disrupt sleep. People who fear nightmares may delay going to bed or use alcohol to achieve sleep, or wake from a nightmare and cannot go back to sleep. They may consciously or unconsciously consider the sleep environment to be threatening, which contributes to insomnia. PTSD is also characterized by physical hyperarousal, which further contributes to insomnia. It is important to address unique factors whenever possible, and may mean treating the comorbid condition before treating the insomnia.

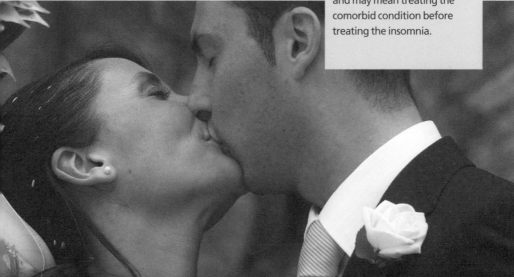

## OTHER TYPES OF INSOMNIA

The following three types of insomnia have symptoms in addition to the general definitions of insomnia.

### PSYCHOPHYSIOLOGICAL INSOMNIA

Psychophysiological insomnia is a disorder in which the person also has evidence of elevated arousal in the bed or bedroom environment and/or evidence of a conditioned sleep difficulty. These can include: an excessive focus on or heightened anxiety about sleep, difficulty in falling asleep when intending to, but an ability to fall asleep in monotonous situations when sleep is not intended, an ability to sleep better away from home, mental arousal in bed, such as intrusive thoughts or the sense that the mind cannot be turned off, and body tension so that it is difficult for the body to relax. Approximately 15 per cent of patients seeking treatment for insomnia have this form.

BELOW *Attempts to get sleep outside of the normal sleep period may seem like a good strategy but could also quickly contribute to difficulty sleeping during the desired period.*

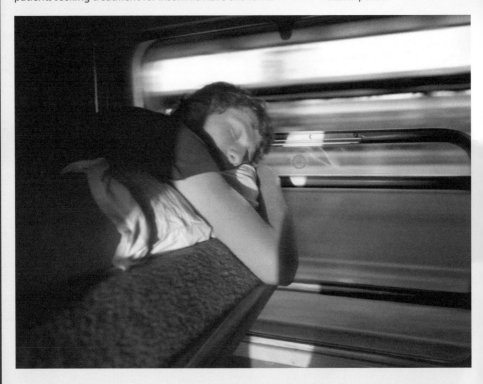

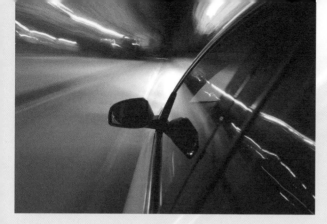

LEFT *Psychophysiological insomnia can be characterized by an ability to fall asleep in monotonous situations, such as being a passenger in a car.*

## PARADOXICAL INSOMNIA

Paradoxical insomnia is a disorder in which the complaint of insomnia and/or non-restorative sleep occurs without objective evidence of a sleep disturbance. Complaints of poor sleep in these individuals appear to be clinically genuine, but objective findings from overnight sleep studies do not reveal sleep disturbances, or the disturbances observed are extremely modest compared with the subjective complaint. There is ongoing debate about whether this form of insomnia may be due to excessive amounts of light sleep and/or multiple brief awakenings that make sufferers feel as though they are not sleeping, when they may, in fact, be in Stages 1 and 2 of sleep. This condition, unlike that of psychophysiological insomnia, requires polysomnography or other objective measures to establish the diagnosis. It is typically found in less than 5 per cent of patients who present for treatment of insomnia.

## IDIOPATHIC INSOMNIA

Idiopathic insomnia is a lifelong and unremitting inability to obtain adequate sleep, which is usually present during infancy and/or childhood and remains through adulthood. Presumably it is due to an abnormality of the neurological control of the sleep–wake system. This disorder may be due to heritable neurochemical imbalances and/or some neuroanatomical abnormalities. While it occurs in less than 1 per cent of the general population, rough estimates are that approximately 10 per cent of patients seeking treatment for insomnia have this idiopathic form.

**More Thoughts on Insomnia**

'People who say they sleep like a baby usually don't have one.'
LEO J. BURKE

'A ruffled mind makes a restless pillow.'
CHARLOTTE BRONTË

'Sleeplessness is a desert without vegetation or inhabitants.'
JESSAMYN WEST

'The worst thing in the world is to try to sleep and not to.'
F. SCOTT FITZGERALD

'For sleep, one needs endless depths of blackness to sink into; daylight is too shallow, it will not cover one.'
ANNE MORROW LINDBERGH

'When you have insomnia, you're never really asleep, and you're never really awake.'
FROM THE FILM *FIGHT CLUB*, BASED ON THE NOVEL BY CHUCK PALAHNIUK

'But no one ever is allowed in Sleepytown, unless he goes to bed in time to take the Sleepytown Express!'
JAMES JACKSON MONTAGUE, *THE SLEEPYTOWN EXPRESS*

## DO SPECIFIC SUBTYPES OF INSOMNIA MATTER?

Whether acute or chronic, primary or comorbid, psychophysiological or idiopathic, insomnia may also present as a specific subtype. These subtypes are based on the nature of the sleep complaint (difficulty in going to sleep, staying asleep or waking too early). The problem of unrefreshing sleep is a fourth subtype. Many sleep researchers believe that the subtype does not particularly matter when we are assessing insomnia, because they all respond well to treatment. However, others take the position that the differences do matter, if we are using an individualized approach with the goal of maximizing the benefits of treatment for each individual with insomnia.

PROBLEMS GETTING TO SLEEP
The person who takes up to an hour to fall asleep on most nights, but sleeps OK after that, has sleep-initiation or sleep-onset insomnia. Such patients tend to be more likely to have features of psycho-physiological insomnia. They report that either their brain or their body remains very active. They may worry about what happened that day or mentally go over their to-do list. Mundane thoughts may also flow through and engage the waking brain instead of allowing the sleep brain

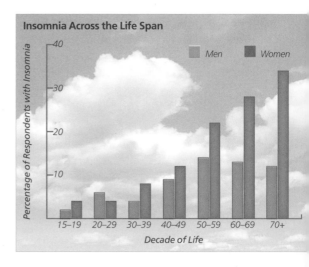

Insomnia Across the Life Span

to function. Such people describe nodding off on the sofa, only to be wide awake when they climb into bed. Body sensations include feeling that the body is tense or energized. These features must be identified and addressed in the individual sleep programme.

## PROBLEMS STAYING ASLEEP

Difficulty staying asleep is also referred to as middle-of-the night or sleep-maintenance insomnia. You will recall that it is normal to briefly wake up a few times per night and return to sleep. It is a mistaken assumption that we 'should' sleep soundly through an entire eight-hour period and waking is only a concern when one or more of those awakenings leads to an extended time awake in the middle of the night.

## UNDERSTANDING SLEEP-MAINTENANCE INSOMNIA

For some people with this kind of insomnia, there may be one long extended wake period, and for others it may be several shorter but still excessive periods of wakefulness. The reader with this insomnia subtype will attest to how distressing this can be, particularly when they followed all the tips and rules of preparing for sleep and fell asleep in a reasonable amount of time. At 2.14 a.m., the digital alarm clock with the red numerals staring back at you is not your friend.

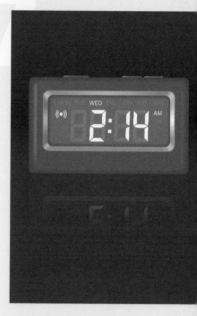

ABOVE *The digital clock is the perfect device to capture our attention and distract us from re-initiating sleep.*

Numbers present the opportunity to do a little sleep arithmetic. 'Let's see. If I go to sleep in the next ten minutes, I will have three more hours to sleep before the alarm goes off. Oh, great, now it's 3.40 a.m., so if I don't fall asleep this second, I'll get under six hours of sleep for the night, and I do not do well on less than six hours. 3.57 a.m. Oh, great…'

Some people who have difficulty staying asleep may have the kind of additional worried thoughts that are present at sleep onset, though this seems to vary. Many people, however, feel as though they are just not tired. This is partly because they may have just had four or more hours of fairly good sleep (including slow-wave sleep that occurs earlier in the night). This can be so pronounced that if it is late enough into the sleep period, people may not feel as if they can go back to sleep at all. Finally, it is important to discern whether the waking pattern is similar each night, or whether it varies from having some good nights, to some bad nights to the occasional horrible night.

## EARLY-MORNING AWAKENINGS

The early-morning-awakening insomnia subtype is characterized by waking early most mornings, often two or more hours before the desired wake time, and being unable to fall back asleep at all. This is often grouped with the difficulty-staying-asleep subtype as sleep-maintenance insomnia. Where it falls in the lexicon of insomnia is, however, irrelevant to the person with this problem. Although it is the least common of the subtypes, it comes with its own frustrations. If the desired wake time is 7 a.m., 4.30 a.m. is awfully early. Staying in bed for two or more hours knowing you are unlikely to sleep is disheartening at best. Some people will choose to get out of bed and start their day. Others find this to be problematic, as it is still dark outside, they do not want to disturb others who may be sleeping, and they think that at least they are resting in bed and will definitely have a zero chance of getting any more sleep if they get up.

This subtype of insomnia seems to occur more often in older adults. It is also the type that may be closest to a circadian-rhythm disorder and, particularly, a phase advance, which has implications for the best treatment approach.

Before moving on, it is important to understand that a person may have more than one of these insomnia subtypes, which is sometimes called 'mixed insomnia'. Nonetheless, it is worth identifying, in detailed fashion, the types and subtypes of insomnia that you are experiencing.

### An Accurate Depiction of Insomnia?

'How do people go to sleep? I'm afraid I've lost the knack. I might try busting myself smartly over the temple with the night-light. I might repeat to myself, slowly and soothingly, a list of quotations beautiful from minds profound; if I can remember any of the damn things.'

DOROTHY PARKER, FROM 'THE LITTLE HOURS' IN *HERE LIES* (1939)

BELOW *Early-morning wakening can be particularly vexing: the mind and body are ready to start the day, but the day has not actually started.*

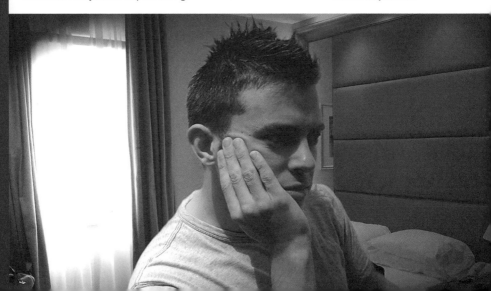

RIGHT *Adequate sleep leads to feeling refreshed. Feeling unrefreshed may be the result of poor quality of sleep rather than inadequate sleep time.*

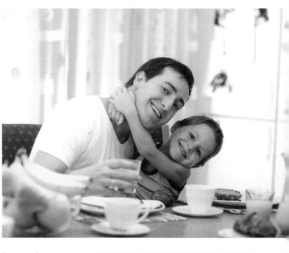

## UNREFRESHING SLEEP

This last insomnia subtype has created a little controversy in the sleep community. Some people find it difficult to understand why someone who does not have sleep-onset or sleep-maintenance insomnia can be said to suffer from insomnia. Others note that there is a subgroup of people who consistently do not feel refreshed when they wake up, and that the problem is not because of any other sleep disorder. Therefore, they argue, it is a sleep disorder in itself and seems most closely related to insomnia. For now it will continue to be viewed as an insomnia subtype.

People with this subtype do have concerns and worries about their sleep and do experience daytime consequences that are similar to those of other insomniacs. There is some suspicion that the quality of their sleep is compromised by either deficiencies in slow-wave sleep and/or an excessive number of very brief awakenings, which may not be registered as awakenings by such people. Possibly this insomnia subtype represents the early phases of the development of one of the other subtypes, although there is currently no data either to deny or bolster this theory.

## A BRIEF SUMMARY

Insomnia comes in a variety of flavours. We are able to group people with insomnia into broad categories like chocolate and vanilla, but, like the offerings of Ben & Jerry's, there are many more distinctive flavours. The major premise of this manual is that the time we devote to identifying your particular insomnia is time well spent.

**An Accurate Depiction of Insomnia – Take 2**

'Now I lay me down not to sleep.

I just get tangled in the sheets.

I swim in sweat three inches deep.

I just lay back and claim defeat...

Lids down, I count sheep. I count heartbeats.

The only thing that counts is that I won't sleep...

My mind is racing, filled with lists of things to do and things I've done.

Another sleepless night's begun...'

FROM 'WHO NEEDS SLEEP?'
BY THE BARE NAKED LADIES

Insomnia can have a number of consequences. This can be measured at both the societal level and the individual level. At the personal level, the effects of insomnia may be subtle or dramatic. What patients with insomnia consistently agree on is that these effects take a toll on them and that they are felt across many domains of their lives. Insomnia is also closely related to a host of medical and mental health conditions. Whether insomnia causes these conditions or the conditions cause insomnia is less important than making sure these conditions are being appropriately managed. The treatments for insomnia that we will review later in this section can be and have been successfully used with positive outcomes, even in the face of some medical and mental health conditions.

# CHAPTER 4
# THE EFFECTS OF INSOMNIA

## QUALITY OF LIFE, HEALTH & WELL-BEING

Just as insomnia may have a variety of causes and may appear in a number of forms, it may also come with quite an array of consequences. Global measures of health and well-being are an attempt to capture the overall effect of the combination of bites that a condition takes out of someone. Generally speaking, insomnia has a negative impact on quality of life. How much of an impact it has varies considerably from person to person, but that impact is far more than a simple nuisance.

### THE PERSONAL EXPERIENCE OF INSOMNIA

A few years ago, sleep researchers at the University of Pittsburgh School of Medicine took a somewhat unique approach to understanding the experience of insomnia. Instead of using surveys or overnight sleep studies, they invited patients with insomnia to join focus groups to respond to and discuss some broad questions about insomnia.

BELOW *In focus group discussions, many insomnia patients insist that their experience of insomnia is quite pervasive across all parts of their lives.*

One salient theme was that insomnia affected all parts of their lives and was not understood by spouses, family, co-workers and treating professionals. Often their doctors assumed insomnia was either 'just stress-related' or diagnosed it as a symptom of depression. The personal experience of insomnia is becoming recognized as a serious problem in its own right by many health-care providers. How they manage or treat insomnia is the next big hurdle.

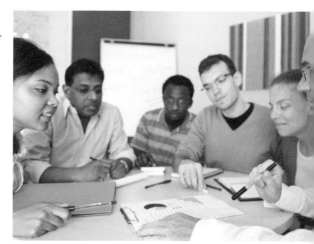

THE IMPACT OF INSOMNIA
Health-related quality of life is often measured with a questionnaire called the SF-36. Thousands of people have completed the SF-36, and anyone who fills it out can be compared with healthy, normal adults as well as with people with specific problems or conditions. In one study, patients with insomnia had pronounced (and negative) differences on each of the questionnaire's eight life domains compared with healthy controls. In another study (Katz and McHorney, 2002), patients with insomnia not only scored 'worse' than healthy controls, but also scored as badly as, or worse than, patients with congestive heart failure.

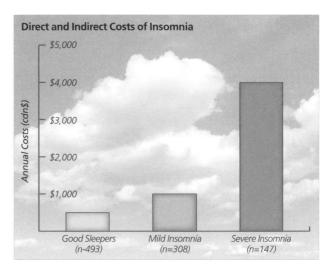

**Direct and Indirect Costs of Insomnia**

Annual Costs (cdn$)

$5,000
$4,000
$3,000
$2,000
$1,000

| Good Sleepers (n-493) | Mild Insomnia (n=308) | Severe Insomnia (n=147) |

CONSEQUENCES OF INSOMNIA
In the United States, health-care costs attributable to insomnia are estimated to exceed $100 billion annually. However, most of these are indirect, and are especially due to motor-vehicle and workplace accidents. Patients with insomnia are two-and-a-half times more likely to report car crashes because of feeling tired than sound sleepers. One study in Australia found that workers with insomnia were eight times more likely to have workplace accidents than good sleepers. These may be indirect costs for government accounting tallies, but they represent real costs to the people involved. Direct health-care costs related to insomnia account for about $13 billion of the $100 billion sum in the United States, because of increased physician visits, prescriptions and medical procedures. A study by Ronald J. Ozminkowski at Cornell University in Ithaca, New York, and colleagues showed that individual health-care expenses of patients with insomnia are $1,200 more per year than those of good sleepers. In a similar study in Canada, insomnia patients spent twice as much on medications per year as their sound-sleeping counterparts.

## FAMILY, SOCIAL & WORK LIFE

One reason why insomnia has such a large impact on overall quality of life is because of the negative effects it can have on people's various life roles. Daytime fatigue and tiredness alone can greatly affect our work, social and family lives.

### SPOUSAL, PARENTAL & FAMILY ROLES

People with chronic insomnia regularly report a decreased ability to handle minor stressors and to be more irritable. A grumpy parent or spouse is no fun to be around. Conversely, people with insomnia also rate their spousal relationships as poorer than those without insomnia. Insomnia sufferers also find decreased enjoyment in family life. For example, the National Sleep Foundation in the United States sponsors an annual 'Sleep in America' poll, which surveys respondents about different aspects of their sleep. One such poll found that those with frequent sleep difficulties rate their ability to function in family and interpersonal roles as poor at higher rates than those with occasional sleep difficulties, and at much higher rates than those with no sleep difficulties.

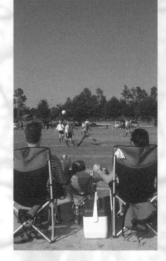

ABOVE *One possible consequence of insomnia is decreased attendance at family activities. Parental duties can be harder to engage in when insomnia is present.*

### SOCIAL ROLES

People with chronic insomnia usually report decreased interest in, and satisfaction from, interpersonal relationships and social interactions. They rate having social disabilities (trouble maintaining their normal social roles) twice as high as those without insomnia. Like many chronic conditions, insomnia reduces the capacity to engage in social activities. Those with insomnia may limit or decrease their social activities because they are too tired to go to the gym in the morning, to attend their child's after-school events, to go out at night, or to entertain friends at home. In addition, insomnia sufferers may get limited sympathy when bringing up sleep difficulties with their friends and may choose to keep their suffering to themselves, even though it has become a prominent part of their lives. This can also diminish the benefits of social interaction.

## WORK ROLES

In terms of work or school performance, chronic insomnia is associated with having less job satisfaction. It is also linked with lower performance scores and productivity. Several studies have also found significantly higher rates of absenteeism in workers with insomnia when compared with good sleepers. Insomniacs report making more errors and having poorer work efficiency than sound sleepers, and workplace accidents are more common in workers with insomnia.

However, I have not encountered many patients who report that work or school absences have increased because of their insomnia. There are few patients who are not concerned about the impact of insomnia on their work performance. Many are also concerned that their generally bad mood negatively affects their family, social and/or workplace relationships. Though few (if any) people become monstrous, even small decrements in role function and a modest deterioration in relationships take a large toll on the individual when multiplied across various life roles. A large multinational study in Europe found that those with severe insomnia were three times more likely to report poor quality of life than those with mild or moderate insomnia, and nine times more likely to do so than those with no sleep difficulties at all.

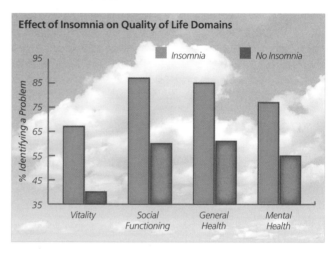

**Effect of Insomnia on Quality of Life Domains**

■ Insomnia   ■ No Insomnia

*% Identifying a Problem*

95 · 85 · 75 · 65 · 55 · 45 · 35

Vitality · Social Functioning · General Health · Mental Health

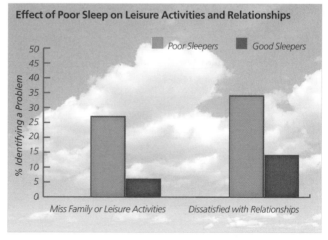

**Effect of Poor Sleep on Leisure Activities and Relationships**

■ Poor Sleepers   ■ Good Sleepers

*% Identifying a Problem*

50 · 45 · 40 · 35 · 30 · 25 · 20 · 15 · 10 · 5 · 0

Miss Family or Leisure Activities · Dissatisfied with Relationships

## MEMORY, CONCENTRATION & LEARNING

We know that sleep loss by itself has an impact on several domains of cognitive function. Researchers believe that the additional features of insomnia, such as hyperarousal, also contribute to such problems. The three main areas of cognitive function that are of concern are alterations in memory, concentration and learning.

## SPECIFIC FINDINGS OF COGNITIVE PERFORMANCE

Numerous studies report that those with insomnia suffer from impaired cognitive performance at higher levels than those without insomnia. People may report an increased level of forgetfulness and difficulty remembering names, common words or phrases. This can be alarming for some and they may be concerned about this being an early sign of cognitive decline. Others report increased difficulty in paying attention for prolonged periods of time, or not being able to read a book without revisiting the same paragraph several times after losing their place. Less commonly, people report feeling as though it is more difficult to learn and retain new material.

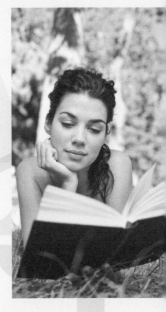

ABOVE *Concentration and the ability to learn new information is negatively impacted by poor sleep and insomnia.*

## PUTTING INSOMNIA & PERFORMANCE TO THE TEST

Studies use various neuropsychological tests, psychomotor tasks (such as attending to a computer screen and responding with key strokes), or vigilance tasks where attention must be maintained. Although in some studies the research subjects with insomnia did far worse than those without insomnia, in other studies few, if any, differences were observed. Researchers in this area have proposed some explanations for these mixed findings. They contend that people with insomnia might focus more on making mistakes or performing poorly than others (or more than they did when they did not have insomnia), so they notice poor performance more often. On the other hand, some have suggested that what the insomniac experiences is an appreciation that extra effort is required to maintain normal or near-normal performance. This latter explanation is congruous with what insomnia patients report when they say they can sometimes maintain function throughout the day, but are wiped out from the effort. For instance, it takes more effort to concentrate when previously little or no effort was required.

## DEPRESSION, ANXIETY & SUBSTANCE ABUSE

Insomnia occurs in 50–80 per cent or more of patients who also suffer from mental-health conditions, such as depression and anxiety. It is so common that insomnia is a recognized symptom in several disorders, including major depression, bipolar disorder, generalized anxiety disorder and post-traumatic stress disorder. The incredibly high prevalence of insomnia in these disorders led to a general conception of insomnia as being 'merely a symptom' of something else. This view – particularly in primary-care medicine and in psychiatry, where great strides have been made to identify and treat depression – resulted in less attention being paid to insomnia as a problem that needed direct attention. Instead, the assumption was that once the 'cause' of insomnia (such as depression) was treated, the insomnia itself would go away. Although this is the outcome for some people, for many others insomnia persists long after the apparent cause has disappeared. Thankfully, this view has begun to change in recent years, which is important because the presence of insomnia puts people at risk of developing a mental-health condition.

## INSOMNIA & DEPRESSION

Having insomnia can be frustrating and depressing. Several common features of insomnia are actually symptoms of depression, such as fatigue or loss of energy, difficulty concentrating or making decisions, and insomnia itself. There is evidence to indicate that full clinical depression and insomnia are closely linked. Both disorders are prevalent and frequently co-occur in all age ranges, especially in older cohorts. You are twice as likely to have insomnia if you are depressed as you are to be clinically depressed if you have insomnia. The co-occurrence of depression and insomnia does not mean that one causes the other, but we do know with certainty that the two disorders are linked.

Beyond that, some believe that insomnia does develop because of depression for some people, and for others depression does occur because of insomnia. The latter assumption has always been difficult for the health-care field to swallow, but there is growing evidence that this can, and does, occur with great frequency.

BELOW *Depression and insomnia represent a chicken-and-egg problem; they are so closely linked that it can be difficult to ascertain which comes first.*

RESEARCH EVALUATING DEPRESSION & INSOMNIA OVER TIME

In a study conducted in patients with a history of having repeated episodes of major depression, the patients were asked to keep track of their depressive symptoms on a weekly basis during a time when they were free from depression. They continued to do this until they experienced a new episode of depression (though some did not develop a new episode during the time of the study). The research team then evaluated the severity of each depressive symptom for each of the weeks leading up to the diagnosed depressive episode. What they found was that insomnia was the first symptom to occur more frequently, and the symptom that was at the highest level of severity at the time the episode began (it was followed by fatigue as a close second). In addition, these elevations were not found in patients who did not have a recurrent episode. This suggests that for these types of patients, the presence of insomnia is a canary in the coal mine, indicating that depression is forthcoming.

Another approach to evaluating the insomnia–depression relationship is to study people who have never suffered from depression, but do have current insomnia. The approach here is to measure the presence of depression at a subsequent point in time. More than a dozen such studies have been published, indicating that those with insomnia have two to four times the risk of developing depression than those without insomnia, measured over the same time period. These time periods are typically between one and three years, although one study evaluated university-aged men over a longer period. For these men, having insomnia in university doubled their risk of developing depression at some point during the following three decades.

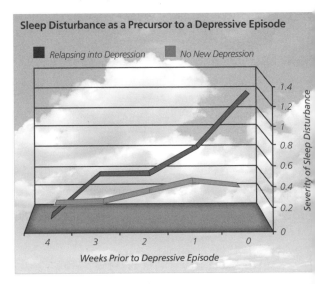

**Sleep Disturbance as a Precursor to a Depressive Episode**

■ *Relapsing into Depression*   ■ *No New Depression*

*Weeks Prior to Depressive Episode*

*Severity of Sleep Disturbance*

1.4 / 1.2 / 1 / 0.8 / 0.6 / 0.4 / 0.2 / 0

4   3   2   1   0

## INSOMNIA & OTHER RELATED CONDITIONS

Insomnia is also associated with bipolar disorder (which is also known as manic depression), and it is well established that insomnia often precedes a manic episode. Complicated grief disorder is not a mood disorder *per se*, but occurs as a reaction to bereavement, the loss of a loved one by death. Between 10 and 20 per cent of people experiencing bereavement have a complicated grief reaction. Difficulty sleeping and/or insomnia has been reported in one-third to half of bereaved people, and at a level of severity higher than in that of nonbereaved people. There is no data, however, that suggest that insomnia is a specific risk factor for complicated grief. There is data, on the other hand, showing that insomnia represents a risk factor for suicide.

## INSOMNIA & ANXIETY DISORDERS

Far less research has been conducted pertaining to insomnia and anxiety disorders, except in post-traumatic stress disorder (PTSD), a severe and often lasting reaction to experiencing or witnessing a traumatic event. The rates of insomnia reach 60–90 per cent in combat veterans with PTSD. However, there is little data to suggest that insomnia contributes directly to PTSD. Instead, we note its high level of prevalence in patients with PTSD, as well as in those who have been exposed to a traumatic event, but may not have PTSD. In addition, insomnia often persists even after PTSD has been successfully treated. This again raises the important point that, regardless of what conditions insomnia may co-occur with, the insomnia itself warrants close attention and probably direct treatment. This also applies to another common disorder, generalized anxiety disorder (GAD), in which insomnia is also frequently observed.

## INSOMNIA & SUBSTANCE-ABUSE DISORDERS

Substance abuse occurs in twice as many individuals with insomnia as it does in those without insomnia. Particularly in alcoholism, insomnia is often reported in the early stages of recovery. It is not uncommon for loss of sleep to contribute to a relapse. In one study, twice as many people with insomnia relapsed within five months of their sobriety date, compared with those without insomnia.

# COMMON MEDICAL DISORDERS

Poor sleep and additional biological factors associated with insomnia can lead to illness. The list of disorders and conditions is long, and is even associated with increased mortality.

### INSOMNIA & CHRONIC PAIN

About half of patients with chronic-pain conditions complain of significant sleep disturbance; some groups have rates as high as 70–88 per cent. There seems to be a two-way relationship between pain and sleep: the worsening of one worsens the other. Poor sleep alone can lead to muscle fatigue and soreness in those with no pre-existing pain, and in the context of existing pain, the effects are quite literally felt. Patients with chronic pain describe waking up repeatedly and not being able to return to sleep – a double blow because sleep is sometimes their only relief from pain.

### INSOMNIA & CARDIOVASCULAR HEALTH

There is growing evidence that insomnia is linked to poor cardio-vascular health. In a study of an annual health-examination database of a Japanese company, over 4,000 men were followed for up to four years, or until they developed hypertension. Difficulty initiating sleep and difficulty maintaining sleep both doubled the men's risk of developing hypertension. A similar study in the US found that difficulty falling asleep, or waking repeatedly, predicted a slightly increased risk of hypertension in about 8,700 participants, while these sleep difficulties, plus waking tired or fatigued, increased the risk of cardio-vascular disease in 11,800 participants by about 50 per cent.

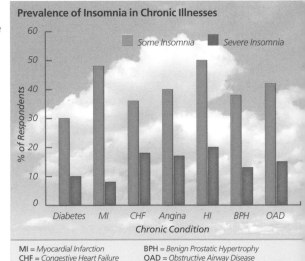

**Prevalence of Insomnia in Chronic Illnesses**

MI = *Myocardial Infarction*
CHF = *Congestive Heart Failure*
HI = *Hip Impairment*
BPH = *Benign Prostatic Hypertrophy*
OAD = *Obstructive Airway Disease*

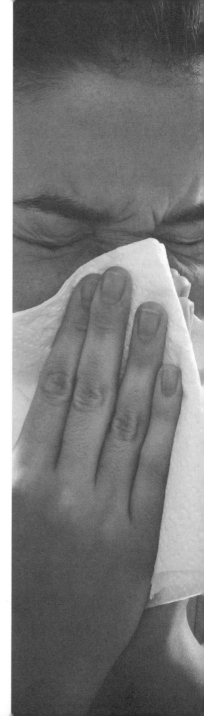

RIGHT *Research shows that people with insomnia are more likely to develop symptoms when they are exposed to the common cold virus.*

## INSOMNIA & OTHER MEDICAL CONDITIONS

Studies have found high rates of sleep disturbance or insomnia in conditions such as gastrointestinal distress, type II diabetes, glucose homeostasis dysregulation (called pre-diabetic syndrome), recovery from cardiac surgery and following chemotherapy for some cancers. Though there is no data to suggest that insomnia causes these conditions, insomnia is often present.

## INSOMNIA & IMMUNE FUNCTION

The immune system is not housed in any one location and has no central organ, but is spread throughout the body. It comprises a vast array of substances that act as a surveillance system. Some substances serve more than one role, and some communicate directly with various brain neurotransmitters. Some of these substances help to regulate the sleep–wake system. The high fever and sleepiness that accompany viral infections such as 'flu, for instance, are adaptive responses to fight the infection that are initiated by the immune system.

Researchers have discovered that levels of immune substances fluctuate during sleep and wake periods, and are altered by sleep loss and sleep deprivation. These include natural killer cells, which attack virus-infected or tumorous cells, and pro-inflammatory cytokines, which amplify the natural inflammation response to injury and infection. These substances are also altered in patients with insomnia compared with good sleepers.

In a study undertaken by Sheldon Cohen and colleagues at the Pittsburgh Mind–Body Center, which was intended to determine whether having strong social connections was protective against the common cold (it was), the researchers observed that having poor sleep quality increased the risk of developing a cold. In 2009, they conducted an experiment to explore this finding. They found that participants with insomnia had higher rates of infection, and that the worse their sleep was, the higher their rates of developing a cold.

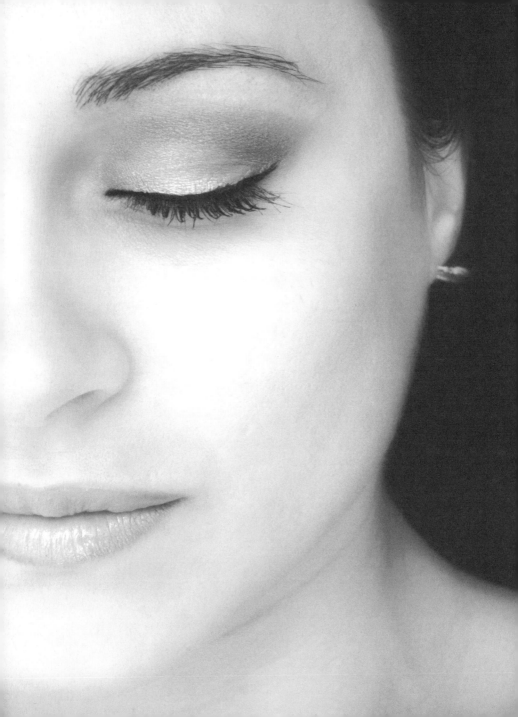

# LEARNING TO SLEEP

The evaluation of your sleep problem that you began in previous chapters takes its final form in this chapter with a thorough assessment of your sleep. This is the last leg in our journey towards identifying your personal brand of insomnia. As you build your own sleep programme, you can begin to lay the foundation for successful sleep by creating a routine that prepares you for sleep and an environment that promotes sleep. This includes both the physical environment of your bedroom and the environment of your mind and body.

# CHAPTER 5
# APPRAISING YOUR SITUATION

## GETTING STARTED:
## EVALUATING AN INSOMNIA PROBLEM

The preceding chapters paved the way for a thorough evaluation of your insomnia problem. I hope you have found at least some examples of your own sleep difficulties within those pages, along with some factors that may have contributed to them. Whenever a sleep specialist who is well versed in treating insomnia first meets a patient, he or she spends a fair amount of time ruling out other possible disorders that may be masking themselves as insomnia – ferreting out all the possible causes of the sleep disturbance, identifying factors that maintain it, and getting a sense of the particular nature and rhythm of the individual's sleep complaints. This is how we will proceed now.

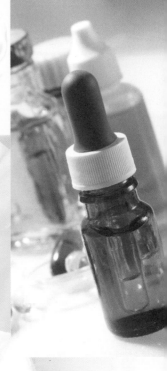

IS THE PROBLEM RELATED TO ANOTHER SLEEP DISORDER?
The first place to start is to make sure that the insomnia is not actually another sleep disorder or primarily caused by one. Sleep apnoea (see page 48) tops this list, because it is a common condition, has significant health consequences and makes treating insomnia extremely difficult. If you regularly snore and are overweight, there is a good chance you may have sleep apnoea. If someone has also observed that your breathing pauses during sleep, then you should get your sleep evaluated in a sleep-disorders centre to determine whether you have sleep apnoea. Once this is treated, if insomnia persists, the approaches in this book can be applied (but not before the apnoea is treated). If you suspect that you may have another sleep disorder described in Chapter 2, it should also be addressed, though insomnia may be treated in conjunction with some of them.

ABOVE *The prescription for your sleep problem will be based on what your evaluation uncovers.*

RIGHT *It is important to take into account any other conditions, such as depression, that are present alongside the insomnia.*

## IS THE PROBLEM RELATED TO ANOTHER MEDICAL OR MENTAL-HEALTH DISORDER?

Insomnia often occurs with other medical or mental-health conditions. If they are being treated, then insomnia treatment may proceed, but discuss the insomnia programme with your health-care providers before commencing. If you have an untreated condition, get it evaluated and treated first. Treatment for insomnia may proceed alongside other treatments.

Are you taking any medications (prescription or over-the-counter), supplements, herbal remedies or other products? Note what you are taking, the dose and when you take it. Next, look at the side-effects list for each medication, and note whether insomnia is listed as a possible side effect. If this is not available, you can do a quick Internet search by typing in the product and 'insomnia' as search terms. If you are taking anything that could potentially be contributing to insomnia, explore other strategies with your doctor.

## A SLEEP HISTORY

Next, create a chronological history of your sleep disturbance. When did it start? If possible, note the time of year. Do you attribute the insomnia to any specific cause at that time? What was going on in your life just then? Were you experiencing any life stressors? Any illnesses? How did the sleep disturbance manifest itself at that time? Note whether you had difficulty falling asleep, if you were waking up repeatedly, being awake for long periods of time at night, waking too early in the morning, waking up feeling unrefreshed from sleep, or some combination of these problems. How long did this last? Did it get better (and if so, how)? When did it return?

Some people struggle with insomnia for many months or years. If this is the case, has the problem changed over time or stayed the same? Has it waxed and waned and if so, what factors may be associated with this pattern? Has insomnia worsened over time, or have its effects on your life changed? Is there any seasonal variation in the insomnia or any other discernible pattern? Have you tried to address your insomnia and if so, how long did you try it for, and what were the results?

> **My Sleep History**
>
> Date insomnia started: . . . . . . . . . . . . . . . . . . . . . . .
> Possible causes: . . . . . . . . . . . . . . . . . . . . . . . . . . . .
> Life circumstances: . . . . . . . . . . . . . . . . . . . . . . . . .
> Nature of problem: . . . . . . . . . . . . . . . . . . . . . . . . . .
> Course over time: . . . . . . . . . . . . . . . . . . . . . . . . . . .
> Patterns: . . . . . . . . . . . . . . . . . . . . . . . . . . . . . . . . . .
> What helps: . . . . . . . . . . . . . . . . . . . . . . . . . . . . . . . .
> What hasn't helped: . . . . . . . . . . . . . . . . . . . . . . . . .

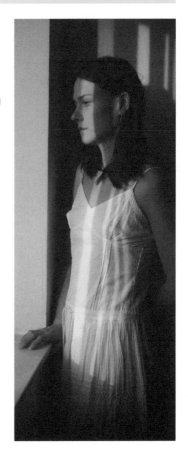

## CURRENT NATURE OF INSOMNIA

Now let us turn to how your current insomnia presents itself. Do you have problems getting to sleep or staying asleep? How often do you wake up and how long does it take you to return to sleep? As your head hits the pillow and the lights go off, how does your body feel? Note whether it feels tired or sore. Is it ready for sleep, or does it seem ready to keep going? Are you too hot or too cold? Similarly, take a survey of your mind at this time. Is it active or ready to drift off to sleep? If it is active, note the kinds of things you are thinking about. Identify any emotions that are present (such as anger, frustration, acceptance, hopelessness, joy). Do the same exercise when you wake during the night.

In addition – although this may vary from week to week – home in on whether sleep problems occur every night and if not, how many nights per week? Identify any patterns to the problem, such as seasonal variations, any relationship with menstrual cycles, or sleeping better on particular days of the week. What might a typical week look like for you? Perhaps two or three bad nights are followed by a good night, and then once in a while there is a dreadfully ugly night.

### Timeline for a Night of Insomnia

|  |  |
|---|---|
| 6.00–8.00 p.m. | Dinner, clean up, chores. |
| 8.00–10.00 p.m. | Family time, catch up on some work. |
| 10.00–11.00 p.m. | Bedtime routine, read in bed. |
| 11.00 p.m. | Lights out. |
| 12.00 a.m. | Still awake, get a snack. |
| 12.30 a.m. | Fall asleep. |
| 2.30 a.m. | Wake up, bathroom, return to sleep. |
| 4.00 a.m. | Wake up, awake for a while. |
| 6.30 a.m. | Wake up, toss and turn. |
| 7.00 a.m. | Get out of bed. |

### The Good, the Bad & the Ugly

Give your sleep a grade of Very Good (VG), Good (G), Bad (B) or Ugly (U). Begin at dinnertime and continue until you get up in the morning. Below is an example from someone who regularly has one really ugly night of sleep per week, interspersed with good and bad nights. Do you notice any other patterns in this example? Carry out this simple tracking of your own sleep pattern for the next two weeks. Do this in conjunction with completing the sleep log on page 113.

| | Sun | Mon | Tues | Wed | Thurs | Fri | Sat |
|---|---|---|---|---|---|---|---|
| Example | B | B | VG | U | B | G | G |
| My Week 1 | | | | | | | |
| My Week 2 | | | | | | | |

## CONSEQUENCES OF INSOMNIA

We also want to identify the daytime consequences that you experience and how insomnia affects your various life roles. Given that an overactive arousal system can be fuelled by stress and can then interfere with sleep, a list of current stressors in your life is required. Finally, it is worth reviewing what factors seem either to exacerbate or ameliorate your insomnia.

**Current Sleep Problems**

Duration of current episode: _____

Description of current sleep problem: _____

Frequency: _____

Patterns: _____

Typical Very Good, Good, Bad and Ugly nights (and frequency of each): _____

What my body feels like: _____

What my mind feels like: _____

Emotions when awake at night: _____

Current stressors: _____

Current medical or mental-health conditions: _____

Current medications: _____

What helps: _____

What hasn't helped: _____

**Daytime Consequences of Insomnia**

*Circle or place a tick beside those consequences that you are experiencing.*

| | |
|---|---|
| Daytime consequences ☐ | Poor role performance ☐ |
| Fatigue or tiredness ☐ | Low school or work productivity ☐ |
| Daytime sleepiness ☐ | Absences from school or work ☐ |
| Low energy ☐ | Making errors ☐ |
| Poor motivation ☐ | Accidents at work ☐ |
| Short attention ☐ | Driving errors or accidents ☐ |
| Poor concentration ☐ | Social inactivity ☐ |
| Poor memory ☐ | Few hobbies and interests ☐ |
| Depressed mood ☐ | Poor family relationships ☐ |
| Irritability ☐ | Worries about sleep ☐ |

## WHAT ARE YOUR SLEEP HABITS?

We want to gather as much information and as precise a set of data as possible with respect to your sleep patterns. This is not only informative, but also will help guide how we address your particular version of insomnia. It will be tempting for you to head straight to the specific treatment recommendations and begin to try some or all of them, but it is very important for you to continue with this thorough investigation.

## HOW KEEPING A SLEEP LOG CAN CLARIFY YOUR SLEEP PROBLEMS

Keeping a sleep log can help shed additional light on the nature of your sleep problems. The sleep log is a daily tally of your sleep over the period of a week. It is suggested that you fill in the sleep log each morning when you start your day, and that you do so for a period of two weeks. Many patients who have not done this before find that, in itself, keeping the log can be somewhat enlightening.

BELOW *A sleep log (or sleep diary) is more graphic or numeric than written, but is also a daily exercise in personal sleep record-keeping.*

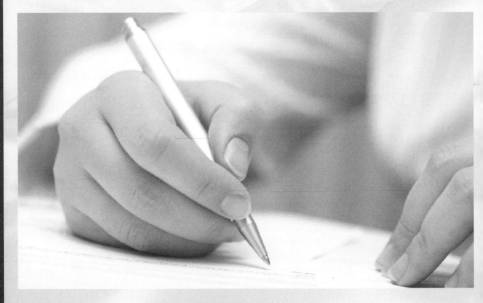

INSTRUCTIONS FOR KEEPING A GRAPHIC SLEEP LOG
Several different versions of sleep logs or diaries have been
constructed, and many of them are available by doing an
Internet search. We will use a graphic sleep log to make this
initial assessment and numerical sleep logs during the active
treatment phase of your sleep programme.

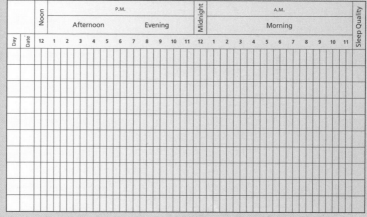

## Example of a Graphic Sleep Log

| Day | Date | Noon | | | | | | | | | | P.M. Afternoon | | | | | | Evening | | | | Midnight | | | | | | A.M. Morning | | | | | | | Sleep Quality |
|-----|------|------|---|---|---|---|---|---|---|---|---|---|---|---|---|---|---|---|---|---|---|---|---|---|---|---|---|---|---|---|---|---|---|---|---|---|
| | | 12 | 1 | 2 | 3 | 4 | 5 | 6 | 7 | 8 | 9 | 10 | 11 | 12 | 1 | 2 | 3 | 4 | 5 | 6 | 7 | 8 | 9 | 10 | 11 | | | |
| F | 3/22 | | | | | | | | | | | | | | | | | | | | | | | | | |
| Sa | 23 | | | | | | | | | | | | | | | | | | | | | | | | | |
| Su | 24 | | | | | | | | | | | | | | | | | | | | | | | | | |
| M | 25 | | | | | | | | | | | | | | | | | | | | | | | | | |
| T | 26 | | | | | | | | | | | | | | | | | | | | | | | | | |
| W | 27 | | | | | | | | | | | | | | | | | | | | | | | | | |
| Th | 28 | | | | | | | | | | | | | | | | | | | | | | | | | |
| F | 29 | | | | | | | | | | | | | | | | | | | | | | | | | |
| Sa | 30 | | | | | | | | | | | | | | | | | | | | | | | | | |
| Su | 31 | | | | | | | | | | | | | | | | | | | | | | | | | |

LEFT *This person's sleep log shows
several afternoon naps and a wide
variability of bedtimes.*

## Your Own Two-week Graphic Sleep Log

**1** Leave awake
periods blank.

**2** Mark bedtimes
with down arrows.

**3** Fill in sleep
periods.

**4** Mark wake-up
times with up
arrows.

**5** Grade the night
as Very Good (VG),
Good (G), Bad (B),
or Ugly (U).

| Day | Date | Noon | | | | | | | | | | P.M. Afternoon | | | | | | Evening | | | | Midnight | | | | | | A.M. Morning | | | | | | | Sleep Quality |
|-----|------|------|---|---|---|---|---|---|---|---|---|---|---|---|---|---|---|---|---|---|---|---|---|---|---|---|---|---|---|---|---|---|---|---|---|---|
| | | 12 | 1 | 2 | 3 | 4 | 5 | 6 | 7 | 8 | 9 | 10 | 11 | 12 | 1 | 2 | 3 | 4 | 5 | 6 | 7 | 8 | 9 | 10 | 11 | | | |

## HOW IS YOUR 'SLEEP HYGIENE'?

While you may not have heard the term 'sleep hygiene', you have undoubtedly seen some version of the sleep tips given opposite (which comprise sleep hygiene) somewhere. You may have even been given a sleep-hygiene handout by a treatment provider. Unfortunately, reading a handout seldom leads to any lasting improvements in sleep. Sleep hygiene is often and widely touted as a wonderful behavioural tool for insomnia, although it has not been found to be effective as a sole treatment for it. Some specialists believe that a list of sleep-hygiene 'dos and don'ts' – in the absence of a more thoughtful and structured approach – not only leads to poor results, but can also dampen enthusiasm for behavioural treatments. When applied correctly, however, sleep hygiene is a useful first step in most insomnia treatment programmes.

## THE PROPER USE OF SLEEP HYGIENE

The concept of sleep hygiene was introduced nearly 100 years ago. The list of tips has grown over the years, but in general includes many commonsense suggestions that can benefit anyone. In the hands of Dr Peter Hauri, the prominent sleep researcher and clinician who popularized the use of sleep hygiene, the treatment was a very involved process. In this structured approach, the patient and clinician review each suggestion in depth, identify those that might pertain to the individual, and negotiate a series of mini-experiments to alter specific sleep-hygiene practices. The patient tracks his or her progress and then reports back on the results.

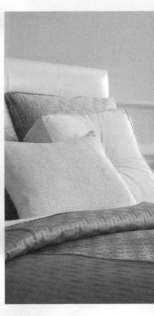

ABOVE *A bedroom that is conducive to sleep is comfortable and free from excess light, noise and temperature extremes.*

When approached in this manner, sleep hygiene can be helpful as part of an overall treatment programme. I consider sleep hygiene to be akin to cleaning and preparing a home workshop before beginning a project, or putting one's desk in order before starting work. In this sense, cleaning up the sleep environment – both in bedrooms and in the way you approach the bedroom – is how we begin treatment. In order to proceed, review the sleep-hygiene instructions opposite, and identify those areas that need 'cleaning'. Even if you have tried one or more of these suggestions before, do please highlight or tick it off.

## Sleep Hygiene Instructions

**1** *Exercise regularly.*

Schedule exercise times so that they do not occur within three hours of when you intend to go to bed. Exercise makes it easier to initiate and deepen sleep.

**2** *Make sure your bedroom is comfortable and free from light and noise.*

A comfortable, noise-free sleep environment will reduce the likelihood that you will wake up during the night. Noise that does not wake you can still disturb the quality of your sleep. Carpeting, insulated curtains, and closing the door may help.

**3** *Make sure your bedroom is at a comfortable temperature at night.*

Excessively warm or cold sleep environments may disturb your sleep.

**4** *Eat regular meals and do not go to bed hungry.*

Hunger can disturb sleep. A light snack at bedtime (especially carbohydrates) may help sleep, but avoid greasy or 'heavy' foods.

**5** *Avoid consuming excessive liquids in the evening.*

Reducing your liquid intake will minimize the need for night-time trips to the bathroom.

**6** *Cut down on all caffeine products.*

Caffeinated beverages and foods (coffee, tea, cola, chocolate) can cause difficulty falling asleep, awakenings during the night and a shallow sleep. Even caffeine in the afternoon can disrupt night-time sleep.

**7** *Avoid alcohol, especially in the evening.*

Although alcohol can help some tense people fall asleep more easily, it also causes awakenings later in the night.

**8** *Smoking may disturb sleep.*

Nicotine is a stimulant. Try not to smoke during the night when you have trouble sleeping.

**9** *Don't take your problems to bed.*

Allocate some time earlier in the evening for working on your problems or planning the next day's activities. Worrying may interfere with initiating sleep and produce a shallow sleep.

**10** *Put the clock under the bed or turn it so that you can't see it.*

Clock-watching can lead to frustration, anger and worry, which all interfere with sleep.

**11** *Avoid naps.*

Staying awake during the day helps you to fall asleep at night.

**12** *Get up at the same time each day, seven days a week.*

A regular wake time in the morning leads to regular times of sleep onset, and also helps to set your 'biological clock'.

# YOUR HEALTH & LIFESTYLE

Here we turn to how your health and lifestyle may contribute to insomnia. This may come in the form of specific stressful events or chronic stress, a range of physical problems, what we put into our brains and bodies, how we care for ourselves, and the myriad of ways in which we get ourselves through the day.

### STRESS & SLEEP

It is widely known that what we call 'stress' has beneficial and negative aspects. A modest amount of stress at important times can help us attend to what needs doing. In extreme situations, what has been called the stress response, or 'fight-or-flight' response, helps us to marshal our internal resources to act quickly to ensure our immediate survival. However, when the stress in our lives is chronically elevated we begin to experience the negative effects of stress in the form of a variety of physical and emotional consequences. Stressful life events are a major cause of new episodes of insomnia, and chronic stress is thought to contribute to chronic insomnia.

Rate your level of stress by answering the questionnaire. Although scales like this are not so precise that one score predicts anything with absolute certainty, there are substantial data to indicate that elevated scores are a good measure of stress levels, so they are a useful way to compare your situation with what others have scored on this scale. If your stress score is elevated, we need to target this in your treatment programme.

### Perceived Stress Scale

### INSTRUCTIONS

The questions in this scale ask you about your feelings and thoughts during the last month. In each case, you will be asked to indicate your response by circling the number representing how often you felt or thought a certain way. Although some of the questions are similar, there are differences between them and you should treat each one as a separate question. The best approach is to answer fairly quickly. That is, don't try to count up the number of times you felt a particular way, but rather indicate the alternative that seems like a reasonable estimate.

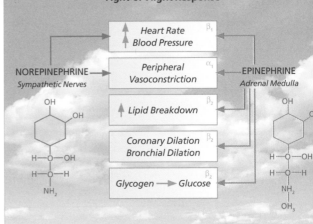

**Fight-or-Flight Response**

| | Never | Almost Never | Sometimes | Fairly Often | Very Often |
|---|---|---|---|---|---|
| **1** In the last month, how often have you been upset because of something that happened unexpectedly? | 0 | 1 | 2 | 3 | 4 |
| **2** In the last month, how often have you felt that you were unable to control the important things in your life? | 0 | 1 | 2 | 3 | 4 |
| **3** In the last month, how often have you felt nervous and 'stressed'? | 0 | 1 | 2 | 3 | 4 |
| **4** In the last month, how often have you felt that things were going your way? | 0 | 1 | 2 | 3 | 4 |
| **5** In the last month, how often have you found that you could not cope with all the things that you had to do? | 0 | 1 | 2 | 3 | 4 |
| **6** In the last month, how often have you been able to control irritations in your life? | 0 | 1 | 2 | 3 | 4 |
| **7** In the last month, how often have you felt that you were on top of things? | 0 | 1 | 2 | 3 | 4 |
| **8** In the last month, how often have you been angered because of things that happened that were outside of your control? | 0 | 1 | 2 | 3 | 4 |
| **9** In the last month, how often have you found yourself thinking about things that you have to accomplish? | 0 | 1 | 2 | 3 | 4 |
| **10** In the last month, how often have you felt that difficulties were piling up so high that you could not overcome them? | 0 | 1 | 2 | 3 | 4 |

**Current Stress Levels**

Score your responses as follows: next to items 1–3, 6 and 9–10 write the number you circled. For items 4, 5, 7 and 8 reverse the scoring (so 0 = 4, 1 = 3, 2 = 2, etc.) and write that number down. Next, add up all ten items to get your total score. If you score above 15 you are considered overstressed.

## ARE PHYSICAL PROBLEMS AFFECTING YOUR SLEEP?

Physical ailments can have a profoundly negative affect on sleep. It bears repeating that any untreated condition should promptly be assessed by your doctor. While some people may have ailments that they feel are not urgent enough to need to see a doctor about – a sore back that comes and goes, or an occasional headache or stomach upset that makes sleep difficult – it may still be worthwhile getting these conditions evaluated. At the very least, they should be added to the list of problems that affect your sleep.

## LIFESTYLE: LOOKING AT DIET & DRUGS

There is not much data to guide us on developing the optimal diet for sleep, but some commonsense tips are available. Foods that are rich in carbohydrates are thought to be helpful for sleep. Most of us have little trouble getting carbohydrates into our diet, though getting them from healthy sources is a bit more challenging. Many diet plans can help you determine what are good carbohydrates, but in general these come from sources such as fruits, potatoes, wholegrain pastas, brown rice and oatmeal. It is also true that the traditional turkey sandwich and glass of milk (or any milk product) can promote sleepiness because of the tryptophan that is available in these foods. Although the science in this area is fairly new and somewhat thin, it is worth considering adding these to your diet if you are lacking in these areas.

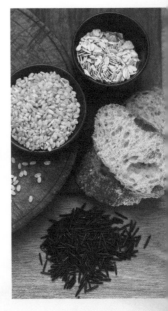

ABOVE *Healthy sources of carbohydrate may play a role in promoting good sleep.*

As the sleep-hygiene instructions specify, both alcohol and tobacco use can create problems with sleep. In general, the use of these substances should be limited in quantity and avoided completely in the several hours preceding your intended bedtime. If this is not already the case for you, then these substances should become the focus for your personal sleep-hygiene plan.

This brings us to the use of caffeine. Some people suggest complete elimination of caffeine, but I fear the global economic fallout of such a practice if everyone with insomnia stopped visiting their favourite coffee shop or energy-drink vendor. Starbucks stock would go into freefall, Mountain Dew and Red Bull would no longer be able to sponsor extreme-sports athletes, and gross domestic product would plummet across the world. I believe a more moderate approach is still helpful for insomnia. Moderate use of caffeine includes one beverage in the morning and another early to mid-afternoon. If you are consuming a lot of caffeine and/or use caffeine into late afternoon and beyond, these practices need to be modified. Finally, be aware of how much caffeine you intake by looking at ingredient lists. Caffeine is measured in milligrams (mg) and is not only present in beverages, but also in dark chocolate and over-the-counter medicines such as headache pills.

CAFFEINE IS A DRUG

In one study, performed by Michael Bonnet and Donna Arand, sound-sleeping subjects who were asked to consume caffeine on a regular basis developed insomnia. Patients often tell me 'coffee does not really affect my sleep', but I always beg to differ. Sleep may come with caffeine still circulating in the body, but a brain on caffeine is far more active and produces lighter sleep than a brain that is caffeine-free. Other people report that they have either cut down on or eliminated the use of caffeine, with no observable difference in their sleep. This shouldn't be doubted, for two reasons. First, since caffeine is a drug, like other drugs it takes a while for the mind and body to acclimatize to its absence, and may even lead to worse insomnia (or certainly increased daytime fatigue and irritability) for a few days or nights. Second, it is unlikely that caffeine is the sole source of your insomnia. Instead, the caffeine needs to be considered as another piece of the insomnia puzzle.

**Caffeine Levels in a Variety of Products**

| Product (all beverages 355 ml) | Caffeine (mg) |
| --- | --- |
| Caffeine tablet (1 tablet regular strength) | 100 |
| Caffeine tablet (1 tablet extra strength) | 200 |
| Excedrin tablet (1 tablet) | 65 |
| Green & Black's Organic Espresso Chocolate Bar (40 g/1½ oz) | 23 |
| Cadbury's Milk Chocolate (28 g/1 oz) | 15 |
| Percolated coffee | 150–250 |
| Drip coffee | 120–320 |
| Coffee, decaffeinated | 10–25 |
| Coffee, espresso | 100 |
| Coffee, Starbucks | 240 |
| Black tea | 100 |
| Green tea | 60 |
| Coca-Cola Classic | 34 |
| Irn Brew | 40 |
| Power Horse | 110 |
| Red Bull | 111 |

## LIFESTYLE: LOOKING AT EXERCISE

Exercise has innumerable benefits and its absence can contribute to poor sleep. Calculate your weekly level of physical activity by noting how long you spend doing modest activity such as walking or moving around, more vigorous aerobic exercise, and anaerobic activities such as lifting materials or strength training. Total the minutes per week and determine the daily average. If your level is less than 90 minutes per week, try adding or increasing regular exercise to your sleep programme (as long as vigorous exercise does not occur closer than 2–3 hours before bedtime).

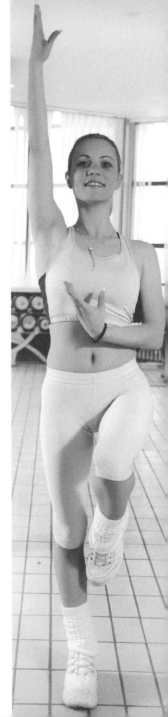

**Weekly Physical Activity**

| *Activity* | *Minutes per Week* |
|---|---|
| Walking | ☐ |
| Running, biking or swimming | ☐ |
| Team or racket sports | ☐ |
| Weight lifting or health-club machines | ☐ |
| Physical work/housework/gardening | ☐ |
| Other | ☐ |
| Total minutes | ☐ |
| Divided by 7 | ☐ |
| Minutes per day | ☐ |

## HOW DAILY ROUTINE AFFECTS HOW YOU SLEEP AT NIGHT

As we continue to look at the flipside of the sleep–life relationship, not only does insomnia lead to daytime consequences, but daytime thoughts and behaviours can also affect sleep at night. We have already noted how this can be the case for stress, caffeine use and exercise. Let's consider a few other examples now.

## THE WEEKDAY ROUTINE

It's 5 a.m. and your four-year-old daughter has just pushed your cat out of your bed, so she can squirm next to you for the next two hours. At the right time, you hit the snooze button on your alarm two or three times. The kids end up getting breakfast at school and you head to the coffee bar again. It's a busy day. You wonder if your restless night of sleep is to blame for your surly disposition. Lunch is from a street vendor (sausage with peppers and onions) and your coffee mug is developing a repetitive strain injury. A chocolate bar and diet coke get you through the afternoon doldrums. Dinner is at the athletic-field snack shack (with a final cup of coffee) while watching your kids' games. Evening is spent paying bills and trying to catch up on the ironing. You finally have a little time to talk (and argue a little) with your spouse once you get to bed.

## THE SUNDAY ROUTINE

The alarm is not set and you sleep in for an extra two hours. Well, you're awake, but don't want to get up. You finally go get some coffee and a bagel, grab the Sunday paper, and head back to bed. Later, a little afternoon television leads to a nap on the sofa. After a late dinner, you realize you haven't prepared for your morning appointment, so you do some work. Just before bedtime you turn on the television to catch the evening news. True to form, a couple of stories get you worked up. Then it's off to bed, wondering if you have prepared enough, deciding you haven't, and setting the alarm for one hour earlier than usual.

## ROUTINES THAT DO NOT PROMOTE SLEEP

The above routines indicate that there is no standard wake-up time – they vary from regular (when you need to get to work early) and flexible (via the snooze button). Kids and pets make poor sleeping partners. Lounging in bed may feel nice, but it sends the wrong message to the sleep–wake system. Coffee in the morning is fine, but a tankful is not. A regular Sunday nap is sure to promote regular Sunday-night insomnia. Late meals, if eaten too close to bedtime, may cause problems. Finally, working and watching the news just before bedtime is not the sleep-friendly evening routine we want to encourage.

LEFT *Regular exercise has been shown to have a beneficial effect on the quality of sleep.*

BELOW *Work schedules can limit the opportunity for sleep during the week, creating sleep debts that get partially repaid during the weekend.*

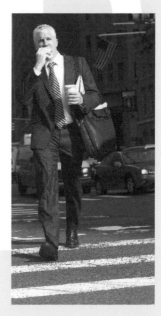

## CREATING A SLEEP SANCTUARY

With the often precise conditions required to promote sleep, and the many large and small factors that can negatively alter sleep, we need to turn our bedrooms into a sleep sanctuary. This requires both a proactive stance to create that sanctuary and a defensive position to guard against disturbances. During the two weeks that you are keeping your daily sleep log, you should complete the myriad of scales, checklists and questionnaires that will guide the development of your sleep programme. The next step in this phase is to identify bedroom-specific factors to address, followed by changes in your daytime and bedtime routines that may be required.

### DETOXIFYING THE BEDROOM

Let's start with the bedroom itself. On the facing page is another checklist to guide this investigation. Identify those items that are currently part of your sleep environment (or are things that you do in bed). As you develop your personal sleep programme in Chapter 8, these items will go on the sleep checklist that will draw on all the checklists you have been creating. It will be up to you to determine which items to target.

At this point, a word of caution is in order. It is natural to look at some of the items and downplay their importance as a contributing factor to your sleep problems. It is equally natural to find it less than appealing to change these items, or to find several reasons why they cannot be changed. You may duly note these objections. At the same time, know that any of these items that are present in your sleep environment are potential pollutants and that you need to have a clean sleep environment. I ask you then to suspend judgement until you have had some time to brainstorm possible solutions to rectifying these sleep-interfering conditions.

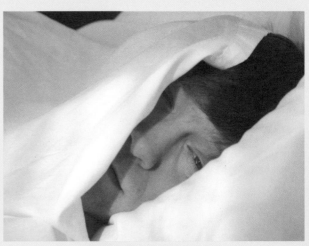

BELOW *Some simple problems such as early morning light entering the bedroom before the desired wake-up time can be easily fixed.*

## Is My Bedroom Conducive to Sleep?

Pets regularly sleep on the bed, in the bedroom or scratch at the door to be let in.

One or more of my children regularly crawls into my bed at some point.

My bed partner or spouse disturbs my sleep with his or her snoring, tossing and turning, reading with the light on, etc.

The room temperature is so cold that I have to sleep with piles of covers.

The room is so warm that I often wake up sweating.

Morning light often wakes me.

My mattress and/or pillows are old and not very comfortable.

I regularly hear neighbours, birds, traffic from outside, and/or creaks, noises and voices from within the home.

I do not feel particularly safe or secure in my home.

There is a television in the bedroom.

I often find myself staring at the clock or repeatedly checking the time.

I read in bed, and often for quite a long time.

I do work in bed.

My bedroom is a staging area for housework such as the ironing pile or for paying bills.

I often have a snack in bed.

## What if I Live in a Studio?

A very real challenge is presented to the person who lives in a one-room dwelling. In this case, the living room, desk and kitchen are literally in your sleep environment. However, many of the sleep-interfering items on the various lists can still be rectified under these circumstances. Essentially, the focus becomes the bed. Any sleep-interfering activities should be removed from the bed. When the bed cannot be physically secluded from the rest of the studio space, by a curtain or other barrier, it is still possible to mentally consider the bed as a separate space that is reserved for your sleep and sex life.

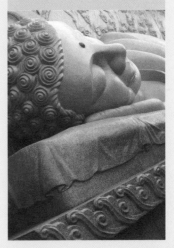

RIGHT *What steps can you take right now to create an environment that is a sanctuary for sleep?*

## DETOXIFYING THE MIND & BODY

Along with detoxifying the sleep environment, you must also attend to your own being. To do so, you need to turn to another checklist, focusing on the state of your mind and body. You will note that most of the items are anchored to the time when you are in bed, although a few items can refer to thoughts or behaviours that may occur throughout the day.

The items that you endorse on this list will help to fine-tune two of the potent strategies that are part of cognitive-behavioural therapy for insomnia. In terms of the mind, many of these items can be addressed as you develop the cognitive-therapy portion of your sleep programme. In terms of the body, a variety of relaxation strategies has proved quite effective (and have mind-calming benefits as well). If you have more than one or two ticks on this list, both of these approaches should be highlighted as you develop potential treatment strategies.

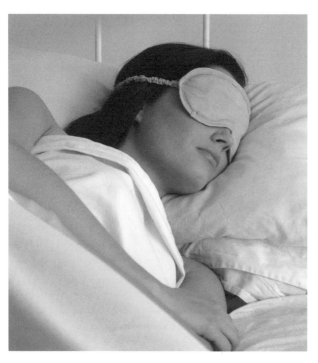

### Matters of Mind & Body

*Of the Mind*
• My partner and I often discuss family issues and problems in bed.
• I do a review of, or think about, the day's events.
• I often do my planning in bed.
• I worry about falling asleep or how I will sleep tonight.
• I worry about how my sleep may affect my day tomorrow.
• I worry about work, family or life problems.
• I feel mentally alert in bed.
• I have difficulty turning off my mind or thoughts.
• I am easily distracted by sounds.

*Of the Body*
• My heart races, pounds or beats irregularly.
• I feel nervous or jittery.
• My body feels electrified or fully alert.
• I feel short of breath or am breathing too fast.
• My muscles feel tight or tense.
• My hands or feet are cold.
• My stomach feels upset or nervous.
• My palms feel sweaty.
• My mouth or throat is dry.

LEFT *Wearing an eye mask is an easy solution to excess light, as are earplugs for blocking out noise.*

## CAN I START A DETOX PROGRAMME RIGHT NOW?

A complete and thorough evaluation of your sleep, sleep habits, sleep patterns and all the potential contributing factors to your sleep problem is under way. Part of this you have been doing mentally, or by completing checklists and questionnaires in this and previous chapters. Hopefully you have also begun to complete the two-week sleep log. When that is finished, you will be able to fully map out a precise profile of your problem and match it to a set of strategies that will make up your sleep programme.

However, there may be some items that you have already identified, feel confident you want to address, and that may take some time to put into practice. For these items the detox process can begin while you are completing your sleep logs. Go back to the checklists and questionnaires that you completed in this chapter. Each item that you want to tackle needs its own plan of action to reach a specified goal. Some will be incredibly straightforward and others more involved. For instance, if the identified problem is clock-watching at night, the goal is some version of 'Don't do that.' The action plan is simply to turn the clock away or place it under your bed. If the problem is that morning light wakes you early, then you need to block the light by installing blackout window blinds or curtains, or by wearing an eye mask while you sleep. These are strategies that you can begin right away.

On the other hand, if the problem is a snoring spouse, a wriggly child who climbs into your bed or a pet that disrupts your sleep, then the goal is clear, but the solution is more involved. For these things, list the possible solutions and the several steps that may be required to reach your goal. It will not take long to develop a detailed plan for arriving at your desired sleep sanctuary.

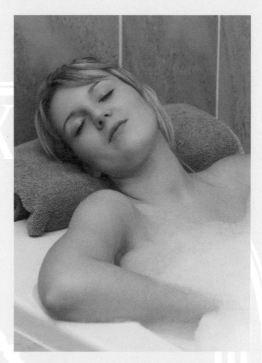

ABOVE *Relaxation approaches are helpful for many conditions, insomnia among them.*

## GETTING MIND & BODY TUNED INTO SLEEP

Detoxifying the bedroom environment is the first step to making a sleep sanctuary. By removing offending items, conditions and practices, the mind and body have far fewer sleep-interfering stimuli to which they can respond. In conjunction with these strategies, the mind and body can also be surrounded with a set of stimuli and conditions that are more sleep-promoting. We want the mind and body to tune into sleep, so that the natural process of sleep can unfold more readily.

### A SLEEP-FRIENDLY ENVIRONMENT

In order to create a sleep sanctuary, all non-sleep items have to be removed. This is a process that can be started now. The television, telephone, laptop, work materials and so on have to find a new home. Some people insist that a television helps them fall asleep. While this may be true some of the time, unless you are falling asleep within 10–15 minutes of the television going on (and it turns off by itself, without waking you up), then it really is not helping you fall asleep, any more than it would if you watched it elsewhere. It has to go. The same logic applies to all other non-sleep items or activities.

Is there something you can add to the bedroom environment to make it more conducive to sleep? Besides light- and noise-reducing strategies, consider what can be done to make the bedroom a more soothing place. Replacing light bulbs with lower-wattage soft light, using high-quality sheets and pillowcases and/or trying a pleasant scent in the room are all possibilities.

### A SLEEP-FRIENDLY ROUTINE

In order to set the stage for sleep, it is helpful to give the mind and body cues that it is time to initiate sleep. The detoxification process removes sleep-interfering behaviours, such as watching the evening news or doing housework or schoolwork up until two minutes before the lights go off, but something must replace these activities. The best way to do this is to evaluate and augment your bedtime routine. Both brain and body need some time to wind down. So start thinking about your bedtime routine not as the five minutes it takes to change into sleepwear and brush your teeth, but as the full hour prior to bedtime.

## AN HOUR OF CALM TO AVOID THE STORM

Tell family, friends and/or co-workers that you will no longer be engaging in sleep-interfering activities past a certain time. This means that any problems that have to be addressed need to be scheduled earlier in the evening or wait until morning. Turn off the television and computer an hour before bedtime, stop doing any physical or mental work, and don't use the phone.

## SOOTHING THE MIND

If you tend to think about your day or problems in bed, do this earlier, within minute three of your last hour before sleeping. In a place other than your bedroom, write out the list of things that you would normally have on your mind at bedtime. For some people, this can be a review and revision of to-do lists. For others, a short diary entry of the day's events is helpful, or it may be helpful to write out the worry list and briefly note the steps already taken (or to be taken) to address the concerns. Whatever written form this takes, leave it on a desk, table or worktop. The unspoken message to yourself is that these thoughts do not need to be taken into the bedroom; they can be picked up in the morning. With the mind temporarily unburdened, engage in a soothing activity next. For some, this can be reading (in a quiet, softly lit room that is not the bedroom). Others may find prayer, meditation or listening to music helpful.

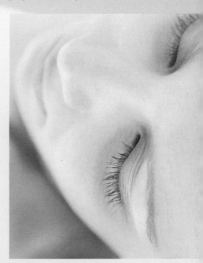

BELOW *The obvious goal of soothing the mind and body is to approach the sleep sanctuary prepared to sleep.*

## SOOTHING THE BODY

To soothe the body, begin by having a light snack. Some activities such as reading or listening to music, can also soothe the body. A hot shower or a warm bath by candlelight are perfect ways to let the body wind down. Warming the body in either way helps the sleep–wake system prepare for sleep by activating a slight body-cooling process that naturally occurs after warming. Also try relaxation techniques, from gentle stretching exercises to guided progressive muscle relaxations.

## THE STAGE IS SET

The stage is set for sleep to occur when a relaxed mind and body enter an environment that is conducive to sleep. Your sleep sanctuary is the setting to enable the powerful sleep strategies in your full sleep programme to work most potently.

There is no shortage of possible treatments for insomnia. These strategies include natural remedies, alternative therapies, cognitive-behavioural therapies, over-the-counter sleep aids and prescription sleep medications. We will explore how these treatments are supposed to work, and their respective advantages and disadvantages. We will also review what the available evidence suggests for the effectiveness of the various treatments within each of these treatment modalities. In this chapter, you can begin to select strategies that you may wish to include in your sleep programme. I would urge you to openly explore all of these potential treatment options. It may well be that the sleep programme that is right for you includes far more than one or two individual strategies.

# CHAPTER 6
# SLEEP TREATMENTS

# NATURAL REMEDIES

A number of naturally occurring substances have been used for the treatment of insomnia. However, the term 'natural remedy' should not be taken to necessarily indicate that a substance is either safe or effective. The claims of success for these remedies are not always matched by scientific support for their safety or efficacy. Here we review some of the more common remedies that have been identified to treat insomnia.

### VALERIAN

Valerian is the name of a plant that has been used as an herbal medicine for centuries. The first mention of its use for insomnia dates back to the Greek physician Galen in the 2nd century A.D. The active ingredient is thought to be from the oil present in the root of the plant (so it is often referred to as 'valerian root'), and the valerian extract is considered a sedative.

As with many remedies extracted from plants, valerian may contain more than one (and sometimes many) active ingredients. One of these ingredients has been shown to interact with brain receptors that are involved in sleep (known as GABA receptors), which are also targeted by many sleep medications. One concern with valerian is that it is sold in several different formulations and recommended dosages range from 75 to 3,000 mg per day.

At least a dozen studies have investigated the use of valerian for sleep, though sleep is not well defined or measured in these studies. Nonetheless, some of the studies have found that valerian improved sleep when compared with a placebo formulation. However, two of the largest studies reported no difference in sleep between valerian and placebo takers. The final word on valerian has yet to be written, and the scientific challenge remains to prove its effectiveness. It may be considered to have possible sleep-promoting effects, with some limited side effects (especially at higher doses), including dizziness, drowsiness, stomach ache, anxiety and night terrors.

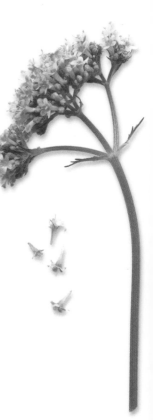

ABOVE *Extracts from the valerian plant have some sedating effect, but have not been shown to improve sleep in insomnia patients compared to a placebo. The current consensus among the sleep community is that valerian is safe, but not particularly effective at treating insomnia.*

## KAVA

Kava is the name of a plant and a beverage derived from the roots of the kava plant. Kava has long been consumed by Pacific cultures for its sedating and relaxing properties. Its many active ingredients have been found to alter GABA-related activity, which may be the basis for its reported effect on sleep. However, there are no studies to support its use as a sleep aid. In fact, although kava seems to have been used safely by Polynesian cultures for centuries, there is clear evidence that kava products can cause liver toxicity and potentially liver damage. For these reasons, kava products are best avoided as a sleep aid.

## TRYPTOPHAN

Tryptophan is an essential amino acid in the human diet and has many uses in the body. One of these is to serve as a precursor for synthesizing the sleep-promoting hormone melatonin. Owing to this, and to the belief that foods that contain tryptophan, such as turkey, are sleep-promoting, several studies have evaluated the effect of tryptophan on sleep. The results have not been convincing. Although turkey does contain tryptophan, it contains no more than other meats. It is now believed that post-Christmas meal drowsiness may be more related to the large intake of carbohydrates and alcohol than to tryptophan.

## MELATONIN

Since melatonin is secreted by the pineal gland and its elevated production aids in the initiation of sleep, it has often been used as a supplement to aid sleep and is perhaps the most widely tested natural substance for sleep. Not all studies using melatonin as a supplement have indicated a positive effect, but some well-designed studies have shown a benefit.

Smaller doses of 1–3 mg of melatonin have proved to be just as beneficial as larger doses. There appear to be no significant side effects when it is used for a brief duration of one to two months. One important caveat: melatonin is much better at shifting sleep rhythms than it is at helping to initiate or maintain sleep. It is possible for someone to take melatonin and make sleep worse. For these reasons, people should not take a prescription for melatonin as a sleep aid unless they have a circadian-rhythm disorder.

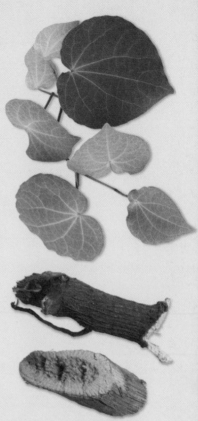

ABOVE *Products made from the kava plant have long been used for their relaxing effect. However, kava can be toxic to the liver and so is best avoided.*

## ALTERNATIVE THERAPIES

Alternative approaches to insomnia have also been used with varying degrees of success. The first set of these approaches has a common goal of achieving a relaxed state that is prepared for sleep. There are many variants and some are no longer considered alternative *per se*. In fact, relaxation techniques in general are often considered an integral part of standard cognitive-behavioural therapy for insomnia. We will review some of the more unique forms of this approach.

### BIOFEEDBACK

Biofeedback is a term to describe a practice in which a constant stream of information about a specific physiological state or function is given to a person, so that he or she may attain some manner of control over this function. This is typically achieved by attaching a sensor to the body that measures a physiological signal then feeds this information back via a computer interface or other electronic device. For instance, an electrode attached to a muscle group can measure muscle tension and give feedback on whether something a person does to relax that muscle can change the signal. This approach has been successfully used to help people reduce muscle tension that contributes to tension headaches. Devices can also measure signals that are related to overall activated (or relaxed) states to teach people to literally alter these states. Once a person has learned how to elicit the desired response, the device is no longer required. However, biofeedback has not been particularly useful in terms of its use for insomnia.

### NEUROFEEDBACK

Neurofeedback is a specific kind of biofeedback that targets control of brain-wave activity. The aim is to achieve a brain-wave state that is conducive to sleep (a relaxed state that precedes

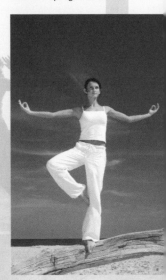

BELOW *Many alternative therapies that promote the relaxation response can be an important component of an insomnia treatment programme.*

sleep and may even include some brain waves that are typically found in light sleep). One of the earliest experiments with neurofeedback was successful in teaching participants to generate brain waves typically seen in Stage 2 sleep, but this did not help them to sleep any better. More recent studies have reported a beneficial effect on sleep.

## YOGA

Yoga is an ancient practice of body and breath control that has been shown to have many health benefits. Any benefits for sleep may be related to the decrease in both mind and body arousal associated with practising yoga. Sleep is often reported as being improved by consistent yoga practice, but few studies have directly measured sleep in patients with insomnia. In one study of 20 participants with insomnia, there was an overall improvement of sleep when they were taught to do a Kundalini form of yoga practice on their own.

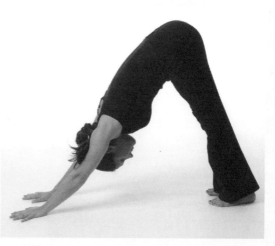

ABOVE *Yoga has been found to improve sleep, and may be a useful technique to include as part of a more comprehensive approach to tackling insomnia.*

## TAI CHI

Like yoga, Tai Chi has a long history of utilization and a similarly long list of beneficial effects. It is considered to be both a light exercise and a slow-moving meditation – thus, like yoga and other similar approaches, it may benefit sleep. A very small handful of studies has demonstrated that Tai Chi can improve sleep quality in those with mild sleep disturbances.

## MEDITATION

The many forms of meditation are also associated with a host of consistently observed health benefits. These are so numerous that meditation should probably be included with exercise and good nutrition as the most powerful tools for sound long-term health. Data on the effects of meditation on good sleep, however, are sparse. Instead of viewing meditation as a single approach for treating insomnia, it may be considered as something that can be added to a multi-pronged programme.

## MORE ALTERNATIVE THERAPIES

The alternative therapies listed here tend to be more passive from the standpoint of the person receiving the therapy. There is very limited evidence for their effect on sleep.

## MASSAGE

Massage can soothe the body and mind, and there is little or any downside to incorporating it into a programme to address insomnia. However, there is no evidence that it improves sleep.

## ACUPUNCTURE

Acupuncture has been used for many health conditions, including insomnia. Specific acupuncture points are used to address insomnia. Although some small studies report beneficial effects on sleep, when acupuncture is compared with another treatment or to a placebo treatment, no improvement in sleep is observed. More and better studies are needed to determine whether it can improve the sleep of people with insomnia.

## HOMOEOPATHY

Homoeopathy, which uses heavily diluted preparations of agents thought to cause effects similar to the symptoms being treated, is similar in concept to the use of vaccines to strengthen the immune system. However, attempts to find the clinical effectiveness of homoeopathy beyond a placebo effect have been unsuccessful. There are homoeopathic remedies for insomnia, but no placebo-controlled trial has tested them.

## AROMATHERAPY

The use of scent from the essential oils of plants to improve mood or health is a small area of alternative medicine. Lavender oil/scent is most often used for insomnia. Two small studies have shown a modest effect of lavender on sleep. However, some oils may cause skin reactions, certain formulations may contain synthetic compounds, and lavender may mimic the effects of oestrogen, so due caution is warranted.

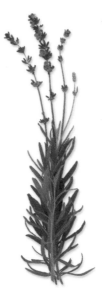

ABOVE *Oil from the lavender plant is often used in aromatherapy, and may help in promoting sleep.*

BELOW *Although massage has not been specifically studied as a sleep aid, it is certainly a good choice for a relaxation strategy.*

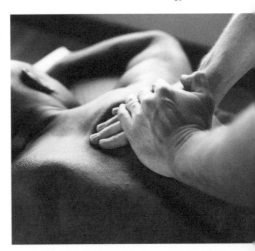

## LIGHT THERAPY

Light therapy uses exposure to sunlight, or to bright light generated by light boxes. This practice is an alternative to standard medications, or to standard behavioural or cognitive approaches to insomnia. Light therapy is best known for the treatment of seasonal affective disorder, where it has been shown to be very effective. It is also an accepted and effective treatment for circadian-rhythm disorders. It is less often used for insomnia, but may be helpful for some specific types.

If your sleep clock has a phase advance (you fall asleep very early and wake very early) or a phase delay (you cannot fall asleep until late at night, but have difficulty waking up in the morning) but it is not severe enough to be classified as a circadian-rhythm disorder, then light exposure may be useful. If you are falling asleep too early, staying up and exposing yourself to bright light in the early evening will shift your clock to a later, more desirable time. Conversely, if your sleep time is already delayed, forcing yourself to wake early and exposing yourself to light in the morning will shift your sleep time to earlier in the night. Note that exposure to sunlight in the middle of the day may be quite healthy and good for your mood, but will have little effect on shifting your sleep clock in one direction or the other.

ABOVE *Exposure to sunlight has a powerful effect on the sleep clock. Light therapy can be helpful in some forms of insomnia.*

## HOW TO USE A LIGHT BOX

Light intensity is measured in lux. Direct sunlight at high noon has an intensity of about 100,000 lux, compared to 100–200 lux in a well-lit room. Light boxes, which can be purchased quite readily, tend to emit light from 2,500 to 10,000 lux (about the same as sunlight at dawn or dusk). If you are using a light box, it should be positioned 45–50 centimetres (18–24 inches) away at approximately eye level. A good rule of thumb is to attempt to expose yourself to the equivalent of 5,000 lux for approximately 30 minutes during the desired periods. This should be done for about one week. If this shifts your clock by the desired amount, you may cure your disorder, though continuing exposure at the same time once in a while will be helpful. Otherwise, if you have shifted about half the desired way back to a normal schedule, shift the timing of your light exposure by that amount and repeat for another week on this new schedule.

## COGNITIVE-BEHAVIOURAL THERAPY

Cognitive-behavioural therapy (CBT) generally refers to a group of strategies used to change thoughts (cognitions) and behaviours that contribute to a particular disorder. Effective CBT treatments exist for a number of common disorders, such as depression, anxiety and chronic pain. All CBT approaches tend to have similar cognitive components, while the behavioural components tend to be more specific to the condition being treated. Typically, all the cognitive and behavioural strategies are used together instead of individually. CBT for insomnia is no exception in this sense, although the behavioural components are very specific to insomnia.

### WHAT ARE THE PIECES OF CBT FOR INSOMNIA?

There are two main types of behavioural strategies in CBT for insomnia. These are called stimulus-control therapy and sleep-restriction therapy. We have also discussed sleep hygiene (see page 114), which can be viewed as a third piece of CBT for insomnia. The fourth piece of the therapy programme is cognitive therapy geared to the thoughts and concerns that are commonly experienced by patients with insomnia. For many people, relaxation therapy or relaxation training, which can be viewed as either a cognitive and/or behavioural strategy, acts as the important fifth element of CBT for insomnia.

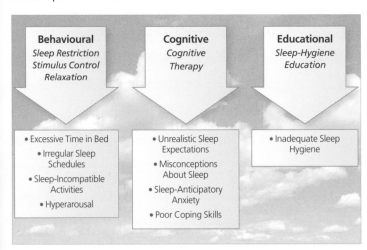

**Behavioural**
*Sleep Restriction*
*Stimulus Control*
*Relaxation*

**Cognitive**
*Cognitive Therapy*

**Educational**
*Sleep-Hygiene Education*

- Excessive Time in Bed
- Irregular Sleep Schedules
- Sleep-Incompatible Activities
- Hyperarousal

- Unrealistic Sleep Expectations
- Misconceptions About Sleep
- Sleep-Anticipatory Anxiety
- Poor Coping Skills

- Inadequate Sleep Hygiene

LEFT *There are three basic types of treatment in CBT, each with a specific purpose.*

## DO I HAVE TO DO ALL THE PIECES?

For most people, it is best to include all the pieces of CBT in their sleep programme. All of the pieces can, and should, be tailored to the individual. It is true that some studies have demonstrated the effectiveness of using single strategies, but most sleep researchers and clinicians recommend that the entire programme be used. The pieces fit nicely together to form a consistent programme that can still be accomplished in just several weeks' time. CBT has proven to be incredibly effective for insomnia when tested in this form.

## HOW & WHY CBT FOR INSOMNIA WORKS

In short, CBT works because, as a whole, the treatments target all the factors that may contribute to insomnia. When the question is 'How does CBT for insomnia work?', the easy answer is 'Very well, thank you.' At this point there are dozens of studies that demonstrate the superiority of CBT for insomnia over all types of control conditions. Several large, well-designed studies have also shown that CBT for insomnia is as effective as (and sometimes superior to) sleep medications in the short term (two months), and better over the longer term. There are very few, if any, side effects of CBT. The most common observation is that some people may actually experience more daytime sleepiness for the first few weeks of treatment. In addition, the sleep-restriction piece of CBT is not recommended for people with a history of mania or seizures, because the sleep-restriction process (which will be explained in detail in the next chapter) may put such people at risk of a manic episode, and sleep deprivation is a known risk factor for seizures. Even for these people, however, the other components of CBT can be employed, and sleep restriction may be modified in such a way that it can safely be utilized.

RIGHT *The interlocking elements of CBT work together to address the many different facets of insomnia.*

### How Drug Names Are Used

Medications have two names: the brand name or trade name under which they are marketed and sold, and the generic name of the drug. For example, Tylenol is the brand name for acetaminophen. In this section, we will follow the convention of calling a drug by its generic name, and putting its brand name in parentheses, as follows: paracetamol (Panadol). Some drugs are sold under a variety of names. For instance, although aspirin was discovered and first sold by the Bayer company, aspirin is sold by other companies. Some drugs have been around for so long that they are allowed to be made and sold under their generic names. That is why we can purchase generic paracetamol rather than the brand-name version. Generic drugs are no different from their brand-named counterparts; they simply use their given names instead.

## SLEEPING PILLS: CAN THEY WORK?

Sleeping pills come in many names and guises. Some can be directly purchased and many more are available by prescription. They can, and do, work for some people, and overall are better at improving sleep than any of the herbal or natural remedies we reviewed. However, most have side effects. Here we explore the pros and cons to help you determine whether a sleep medication should be part of your sleep programme.

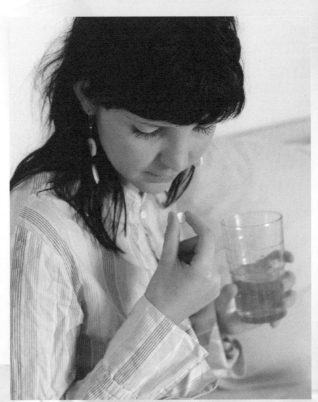

RIGHT *Both over-the-counter and prescription sleep aids can improve the sleep of people with insomnia.*

## OVER-THE-COUNTER MEDICATIONS

The many over-the-counter medications (referred to as OTCs) for sleep, but as always you should discuss any medications with your doctor or other qualified medical professional before embarking on any course of medications. In particular, brand names tend to change, or vary between countries, so do check this with your doctor and/or your pharmacist. The following information, therefore, is here just as a guide.

Diphenhydramine, is the most common active ingredient in OTC sleep aids. In many brand-name sleep aids, this drug is combined with paracetamol. The second variety of OTC sleep aids is doxylamine, which is also combined with paracetamol.

Interesting, the active ingredients in OTC sleep aids are often the same as those found in some OTC allergy medications that are sedating anti-histamines. Furthermore, the main side effect of these types of antihistamine drugs (e.g. promethazine) is drowsiness. Most OTC sleep aids, then, are based on drowsiness as a side effect of these types of antihistamines. Histamines, which are naturally produced by the body, promote wakefulness; antihistamines block this process and result in drowsiness. OTC sleep aids do have side effects, including daytime drowsiness, dry mouth and dizziness. They are to be avoided by people with kidney or liver disease, glaucoma or prostate or urination problems.

The sleep-promoting effects of these OTCs do not last long. After just a few days, they fail to help sleep altogether. If they are used, therefore, it should be only for a night or two.

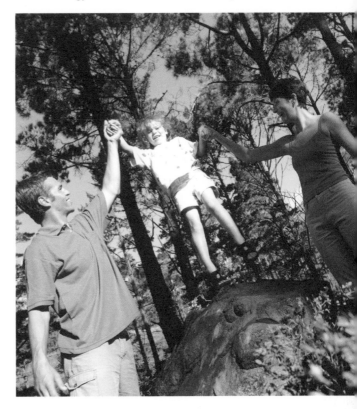

BELOW *Daytime drowsiness is a common side effect of many over-the-counter medications for sleep, so try to avoid taking them if you need to be particularly alert and wakeful for a daytime event.*

## PRESCRIPTION MEDICATIONS

There are several different types of prescription sleep medications, although they are all considered to be sedative hypnotic medications. They generally work by interacting with brain receptors that are involved in the regulation of sleep. Some of these medications have been around for decades, while others were introduced to the marketplace more recently. In the UK, the National Institute for Health and Clinical Excellence (NICE), the organization that provides guidance on new and existing medications, has approved zaleplon, zolpidem and zopiclone. Other drugs are in various stages of testing, and there are others used for insomnia although they do not have specific indications for treating the disorder.

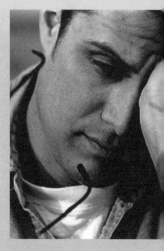

ABOVE *Sleep medications with longer half lives can cause morning drowsiness. Some people call this the 'hangover effect'.*

### Half-Lives of Sleep Medications

All medications have a specific amount of time that they remain active in the body. This is often measured in terms of the drug's half-life (the time it takes for half of the medication to be metabolized). The longer the half-life, the longer the medication is active in the body. This is important because medications with very long half-lives may still be active in the body after someone wakes up, leading to daytime sedation or drowsiness. On the other hand, a medication with a very short half-life may only work for a brief period of time.

| Drug | Half-Life (in hours) |
| --- | --- |
| Flurazepam | 48–120 |
| Temazepam | 8–20 |
| Triazolam | 2–6 |
| Estazolam | 8–24 |
| Quazepam | 48–120 |
| Zolpidem | 1.5–2.4 |
| Zaleplon | 1 |
| Zopiclone | 5–7 |

## BENZODIAZEPINE SEDATIVE HYPNOTICS

Benzodiazepines are the oldest class of sleep medications of the drugs marketed as sedative hypnotics. These prescription drugs include estazolam, flurazepam, quazepam, temazepam and triazolam. In general, these medications are considered to be effective in treating insomnia, but they have more serious side effects than some of the newer sleep medications. In particular, these benzodiazepines have a risk of tolerance building (needing more medication to achieve the same effect) and dependence. Their fairly long half-lives mean they are more likely to cause daytime sedation and are associated with injuries from falls, especially in the elderly.

## NON-BENZODIAZEPINE, BENZODIAZEPINE RECEPTOR AGONIST SEDATIVE HYPNOTICS

The BZRAs (as these are called for short) are a newer class of medications with the same chemical structure, and acting on the same brain receptors as benzodiazepines, but they act a little more precisely. They include zopiclone, zaleplon and zolpidem. They have shorter half-lives than benzodiazepines, are thought to have fewer side effects and less risk of dependency, but are still considered controlled substances. All of these medications have proven effectiveness for insomnia that includes sleep-onset problems.

Common side effects for this class of medications can include headache, dizziness, dry mouth and infections, with more rare reports of allergic reactions, facial swelling, complex sleep-related behaviours (such as driving or eating with no recall of the event), memory lapses and hallucinations. Zopiclone is also effective for sleep-maintenance insomnia.

## MELATONIN RECEPTOR AGONIST HYPNOTIC

Although not currently approved for use in the UK, it is worth noting that ramelteon is a unique medication that acts on melatonin receptors. This medication mimics the sleep-regulation hormone melatonin and has also been shown to be effective for sleep-onset problems and not as effective for problems in staying asleep. It is not a controlled substance, has little or no risk of physical dependency, but does have some limited side effects.

BELOW *Some hypnotic medications, particularly the benzodiazepines, are associated with injuries from falls in older adults.*

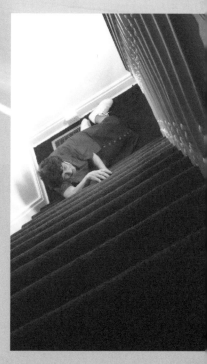

## WHICH SLEEP MEDICATION IS RIGHT FOR ME?

As you can see, there are many sleep medication options to choose from. The decision about which sleep medication to try will depend on whether your current insomnia episode began very recently or has been ongoing for one or more months. It will also depend on whether you primarily have difficulty staying asleep, falling asleep or both. I suggest that there is little reason to consider any of the benzodiazepine medications, and will remind you that OTC sleep aids are only useful for one or two nights. That leaves five sleep medications to consider for longer-term use.

### THE 'Z' DRUGS & RAMELTEON

Zopiclone, zaleplon and zolpidem are sometimes referred to as the 'Z' drugs and, combined with ramelteon, represent the best choices for insomnia treatment. Any of these medications can be considered if the insomnia is mainly related to problems falling asleep.

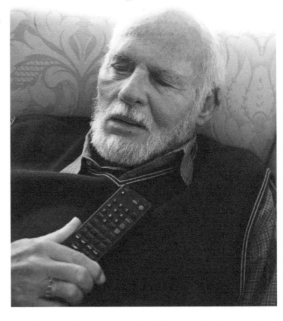

ABOVE *Sleep medications can act quickly; it is best to take them as part of your pre-bedtime routine.*

Zaleplon in particular is especially useful if your main problem is falling asleep, since it has an extremely short half-life and is out of your system well before you wake up in the morning. Zopiclone is the best choice for insomnia that includes middle-of-the-night awakenings and/or sleep-maintenance problems. Since it has a short half-life, zaleplon (in consultation with a prescribing doctor) may also be taken in the middle of the night if there are at least four or five hours remaining before your desired wake time. Although not yet approved in the UK, ramelteon is considered to be the safest sleep medication in the United States, with the smallest number of potential side effects if consequences are a concern.

## HOW LONG TO TAKE A SLEEP MEDICATION

If you have very recently developed insomnia, this may be a good time to try a sleep medication for a brief period of 7–10 days. Although CBT strategies should also be used, these tend to take longer to work, so a sleep medication may help prevent the development of chronic insomnia. The standard recommended duration of treatment using sleep medication for insomnia that is already chronic is 28 days. Of course, many people take medications for several months, or even years. However, we do not know how safe and effective it is to use sleep medications for years on end. We do, though, have good data that the 'Z' drugs are safe and effective for as long as six months. Presumably, however, one of the reasons you are reading this manual is to avoid or discontinue using medications.

## COMBINING SLEEPING PILLS WITH OTHER APPROACHES

Some work has been directed at both helping people to discontinue use of sleep medications and/or at helping them to combine them with CBT approaches. Charles Morin and his colleagues at the University of Laval in Quebec have shown that CBT can be successfully combined with sleep medication in a programme where the sleep medication is gradually discontinued during the course of CBT. Interestingly, they found that people who discontinued their medication did better over the long term than those who continued to use sleep medications, even though they had also received CBT. If you feel that you need a sleep medication to begin your treatment programme, or if you are currently on a sleep medication, then designing and building a withdrawal schedule into your sleep programme makes good sense. This can either be initiated 3–4 weeks into your treatment programme or near its conclusion. A useful withdrawal (or taper) schedule is to take half the dose of the medication nightly for one week and then to continue taking this reduced amount on an every-other-night schedule for 1–2 weeks, before completely stopping its use.

### Considerations for Any Sleep Medication

• Inform your doctor about other medications that you are taking, including non-prescription or OTC medications and herbal remedies or supplements.

• Likewise, inform your doctor of other medical conditions that you have, to avoid serious side effects.

• Follow the directions closely, which usually means starting with a small dose of the medication and increasing it gradually, according to the doctor's schedule.

• For the best effect, take the medication approximately 30 minutes before your desired bedtime.

• Never drink alcohol near the time when you take a sleeping pill, and never drive a car or operate machinery after taking a sleeping pill.

• Ask your doctor for specific instructions for decreasing and/or discontinuing the medication's use.

This sleep workshop is an intimate and very detailed 'how-to' guide for implanting the core features of a cognitive-behavioural therapy programme for insomnia. Of all the treatment strategies reviewed in the previous chapter, the cognitive behavioural approach is the most demanding. It also happens to be the most successful approach for managing insomnia. Using cognitive-behavioural strategies does not preclude any of the other treatment strategies. I do suggest for most people, however, that it serves as a cornerstone of a complete programme. In this chapter, we will walk through the steps that will lead to the successful application of the cognitive and behavioural practices that lead to improved sleep.

# CHAPTER 7
# SLEEP WORKSHOP

# START WITH A SLEEP LOG

Hopefully, the graphic sleep log (see page 112) that you have kept, or are keeping, will provide some insight into your sleep patterns. You should continue to keep a daily sleep log throughout the entire length of your sleep programme, although this will be a numerical sleep log.

## WHY SLEEP EXPERTS RECOMMEND KEEPING A SLEEP LOG

There are four very good reasons to keep daily sleep logs consistently and accurately. First, they can continue to provide valuable information about your sleep patterns and how these change with each phase of treatment. Second, the very act of recording the data can lead to better sleep habits as you engage in this low-tech version of biofeedback. Third, sleep-restriction therapy (which is a critical part of CBT) depends on precise data from your sleep logs in order to make weekly changes in your prescribed sleep schedule. Finally, by calculating the weekly averages of several sleep variables derived from the sleep logs, you can plot how these variables are changing over time. This can be very encouraging and serves to reinforce the positive changes that you are making to improve your sleep.

## SAMPLE SLEEP LOG TO ADAPT FOR YOUR OWN USE

Opposite is a sample of a numerical sleep log to be used over a one-week period. Part I of the sleep log (the top half) is just a sample of the things you may want to record. You can use it as is, ignore it completely or add and delete items as you see fit. Part II of the sleep log is not adjustable. Here you enter the values as directed opposite. The spreadsheet will calculate weekly averages for you to plot on a graph.

RIGHT *This is an example of a one-week numerical sleep log, with the first night filled out as a guide to help you fill out your own.*

FAR RIGHT *A trip to the refrigerator would be captured on the sleep log under 'Minutes out of bed while awake during the night'.*

## Tips for Completing the Sleep Log

• Except for your bedtime and the time you get up in the morning, avoid looking at the clock to get exact numbers for the other variables. A good estimate will suffice for minutes to fall asleep and the number of times you wake up. Also, do not try to keep mental notes of these times during the night (or turn a light on to write the numbers down). Just estimate the values when you fill out your sleep log in the morning.

• 'Minutes awake after you first fell asleep' refers to the length of time it took you to fall back to sleep after you had woken up during the night. Let's assume someone went to bed at 12.30 a.m., fell asleep at 12.45 a.m., woke up for 10 minutes at 2.00 a.m., then woke up again at 3.30 a.m., taking 30 minutes to fall back asleep. They remained asleep until five minutes before they got up at 6.30 a.m. On the sleep log, we have added the 10- and 30-minute awakenings together and entered these as two awakenings lasting 40 minutes. The final awakening of five minutes gets its own line.

• 'Minutes out of bed while awake during the night' is used to count the time out of bed for things such as bathroom runs and snack breaks. Sleep efficiency is a percentage that is calculated by dividing the total sleep time for the night by the total sleep period. In our example on the sleep log, this was 300 minutes divided by 360 minutes (or about 83 per cent).

### COMPLETE IMMEDIATELY UPON AWAKENING

| Date | Example Monday | | | | | | | Weekly Average |
|---|---|---|---|---|---|---|---|---|
| Time to bed | 12.30 a.m. | | | | | | | |
| Time out of bed for the day | 6.30 a.m. | | | | | | | |
| Minutes to fall asleep | 15 | | | | | | | |
| Times You woke up | 2 | | | | | | | |
| Minutes awake after you first fell asleep | 40 | | | | | | | |
| On your last awakening before getting out of bed, how many minutes were you awake? | 5 | | | | | | | |
| Minutes out of bed while awake during the night | 0 | | | | | | | |
| Total sleep time (minutes) | 300 | | | | | | | |
| Sleep efficiency % (Total sleep time/time in bed) | 83% | | | | | | | |

## STIMULUS-CONTROL THERAPY

Stimulus-control therapy for insomnia was first developed by Richard Bootzin at the University of Arizona in the early 1970s. It has been widely evaluated as both a single therapy and as part of CBT, where it is considered an integral part of a multi-strategy approach to insomnia. The therapy is based on very sound principles of how insomnia develops and is maintained by environmental and behavioural factors. The instructions are straightforward but their implementation can be challenging.

### HOW STIMULUS CONTROL WORKS

Stimulus-control instructions are based on a theoretical model of insomnia that explains the development and maintenance of insomnia as being partly due to learning or conditioning. You may recall from a sixth-form college or university biology or psychology course that conditioning may occur when a behaviour is repeatedly paired with one or more stimuli in the environment, such that the mere presence of those stimuli can come to elicit the behaviour on its own. The classic example of this phenomenon is Pavlov's dogs. Dr Ivan Pavlov's dogs salivated whenever food was presented. The presentation of food was paired with an auditory tone. Over time, the dogs salivated on hearing the tone, although no food was presented. Drooling became a conditioned response to the tone.

With respect to insomnia, the bedroom environment becomes paired with all manner of stimuli that are present while the person with insomnia struggles awake in bed for many nights. Over time, merely entering the bedroom environment or getting into bed elicits a physical and cognitive arousal response. Thus, for some people, insomnia is partly related to conditioned arousal brought forth by the bedroom environment.

The goals of stimulus-control therapy are to rectify this situation by strengthening the bed and bedroom as cues for sleep and weakening them as cues for arousal, while developing a consistent sleep–wake schedule as a time cue for sleep.

INSTRUCTIONS & IMPLEMENTATION
Stimulus-control instructions include: (1) keeping a fixed wake time seven days per week, irrespective of how much sleep you get during the night; (2) avoiding any behaviour in the bed or bedroom other than sleep or sexual activity; (3) leaving the bedroom when awake for 15 minutes or so; (4) going to bed only when sleepy.

Most people find the most difficult facet of stimulus control is having to leave the bedroom if they are awake for more than 15 minutes. This means that you must physically get out of bed and go elsewhere – including if you are awake after first going to bed, or (more challenging) if you are awake in the middle of the night. Most people find the best thing to do is to engage in a sedentary and/or soothing activity such as reading. You should not return to bed until you are sleepy and you may find that you have to repeat the process more than once on some nights.

*BELOW Stimulus control requires that the bed and the bedroom be used almost exclusively for sleeping and for sex. Developing a consistent sleep–wake schedule as a cue for sleep tends to help train the circadian sleep–wake cycle to the desired phase.*

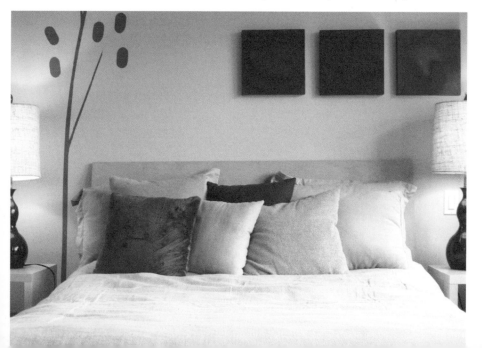

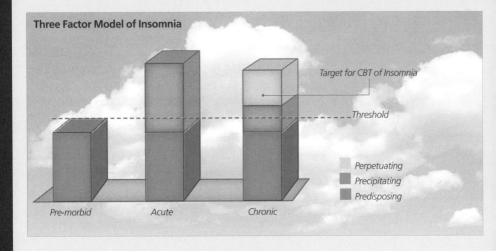

**Three Factor Model of Insomnia**

Target for CBT of Insomnia

Threshold

Perpetuating
Precipitating
Predisposing

Pre-morbid   Acute   Chronic

## SLEEP-RESTRICTION THERAPY

Sleep-restriction therapy was developed by Art Spielman and colleagues in the mid-1980s at the City University of New York. It is based on his theoretical model of insomnia, which recognizes that insomnia may be caused by one set of factors, but that it is partially maintained by what he called 'perpetuating factors'. These were based on observations that people with insomnia tend to engage in behaviours that may make sense, but serve to tighten rather than loosen the hold of insomnia. Sleep restriction endeavours to reverse this process.

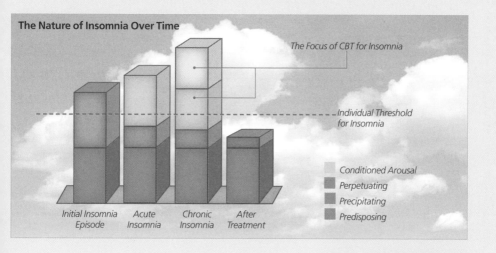

**The Nature of Insomnia Over Time**

The Focus of CBT for Insomnia

Individual Threshold
for Insomnia

Conditioned Arousal
Perpetuating
Precipitating
Predisposing

| Initial Insomnia Episode | Acute Insomnia | Chronic Insomnia | After Treatment |

## HOW SLEEP RESTRICTION WORKS

The perpetuating factors that Dr Spielman recognized include maladaptive strategies adopted in an attempt to get more sleep or recover from sleep loss. For instance, someone may go to bed earlier than usual or get out of bed later in order to increase the opportunity to get more sleep. Unfortunately, when the opportunity to sleep exceeds the brain and body's ability to generate sleep, the consequence is more frequent and longer awakenings. In addition, people may stay in bed while awake for long periods of time, either to increase the likelihood of getting more sleep or with the mistaken assumption that staying in bed is at least 'restful'.

While this is seemingly reasonable behaviour, staying in bed while awake leads to an association of the bed and bedroom with arousal, not with sleepiness and sleep. The two maladaptive behaviours (extending sleep opportunity and staying in bed when awake) are likely to occur together and promote one another. Excessive time in bed increases the likelihood that you will be awake while in bed. Being awake in bed, meanwhile, increases the likelihood that you will attempt to get more sleep by increasing your sleep opportunity. Sleep restriction essentially addresses the mismatch between your sleep opportunity and your sleep ability.

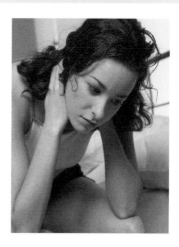

ABOVE *Sleep restriction works by creating sleepiness at the appropriate time – in other words, when you go to bed.*

## INSTRUCTIONS & IMPLEMENTATION

Sleep restriction addresses the mismatch between sleep opportunity and ability by limiting the amount of time that you spend in bed. In this regard it works hand-in-hand with stimulus control. However, sleep restriction goes a step further by rigidly fixing your actual bedtimes and rise times. First, you start by establishing a fixed wake time. This may be your preferred wake time, or the time you need to get up to start your day without being excessively rushed. If your insomnia is such that you almost always wake up (and stay awake) two hours before your desired wake time, you can split the difference. In other words, if you desire to wake at 7.00 a.m., but habitually wake at 5.00 a.m., you can set your wake time as 6.00 a.m.

## ESTABLISHING A SLEEP WINDOW

With a wake time established, you need your weekly average total sleep time from your numerical sleep log. Continuing with our example, if your total average sleep time is 5$\frac{1}{2}$ hours, you want to set your bedtime 5$\frac{1}{2}$ hours from your 6.00 a.m. wake time. Your 'sleep window', then, is 12.30–6.00 a.m. This schedule is to be maintained during weekdays and weekends. One important caveat in establishing your sleep window is never to set it smaller than 5 hours, even if your average sleep time is less than 5 hours.

Initially, the therapy may result in a reduction in total sleep time, but over the course of several days will result in decreased time to fall asleep and decreased time awake in the middle of the night. As a result, your sleep efficiency will increase. Importantly, you may not feel any different (and may even feel more tired) because your total sleep time is limited to 5$\frac{1}{2}$ hours a night at most. If this were all there were to sleep restriction, it would not be sustainable.

## ADJUSTING YOUR SLEEP WINDOW

As your sleep efficiency increases and is sustained at these higher levels, however, you can gradually widen your sleep window. This is done according to a formula driven by your sleep logs. On a weekly basis, you can increase the amount of time spent in bed in 15-minute increments. For most people, it is optimal to extend the sleep window by keeping the morning wake time the same, but making bedtime 15 minutes earlier.

The formula for when to extend the sleep window is based on your average sleep efficiency for one week. Recall that sleep efficiency is calculated by taking your average total sleep time for the week and dividing it by your sleep window (in minutes). If your sleep efficiency for the week is 90 per cent or more, then increase your sleep window by 15 minutes (otherwise the sleep window is unchanged). This process continues on a weekly basis until you arrive at a sleep window that allows for an adequate amount of sleep and still maintains sleep efficiency above 90 percent.

THE EVENTUAL GAIN IS WORTH THE INITIAL PAIN
Sleep restriction works on several features of insomnia. By preventing the practice of stretching sleep opportunity over too long a period, the sleep you get is more consolidated and less fragmented. In addition, it is thought to increase the 'pressure for sleep', which helps to rebalance sleep homeostasis. The regular bed and wake times, in turn, help to align your sleep clock. Finally, like stimulus control, sleep restriction weakens associations between the bedroom and being awake because most of your time in bed will be taken up with sleep.

BELOW *Sleep restriction can be difficult to initiate, but this approach consistently leads insomnia patients to better sleep.*

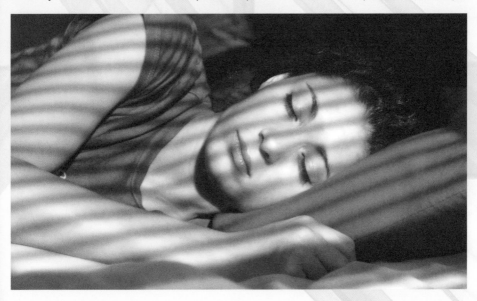

## COGNITIVE THERAPY

Cognitive therapy was largely brought to use for the treatment of insomnia through the efforts of Charles Morin in the late 1980s and early 1990s, and has since been refined and expanded by other prominent sleep researchers and clinicians. In general, cognitive therapy, when used for insomnia, is based on the observation that patients with insomnia have negative thoughts and beliefs about their condition and its consequences, which may be well warranted but are more harmful than useful. The goal of cognitive therapy is to reduce or eliminate these unhelpful thoughts or beliefs. In so doing, they are removed from the combination of factors contributing to insomnia.

### HOW COGNITIVE THERAPY WORKS

Cognitive therapy, like the other approaches in CBT, is seemingly straightforward. It begins by assessing some of the common thoughts and beliefs that hinder a more useful attitude towards sleep. Cognitive therapy targets these thoughts, which can often be automatic. To begin assessing some of your thoughts, check off those beliefs you sometimes have that are listed opposite. You may want to highlight those thoughts or beliefs that are particularly strong or frequent.

## How My Thoughts Hinder My Sleep

• When I don't get a proper amount of sleep on a given night, I need to catch up by napping the next day or by going to bed earlier the following night.

• I need eight hours of sleep to function properly.

• I worry that if I go for one or two nights without adequate sleep I could completely 'fall apart'.

• I worry that chronic insomnia could have serious consequences for my physical health.

• When I have trouble falling asleep, my feeling is that I should stay in bed because I might fall asleep, or at the very least I'll get some rest.

• When I have trouble getting to sleep, I should stay in bed and try harder.

• I worry that I might lose control over my ability to sleep.

• After a poor night's sleep, I know that my ability to function the next day will be compromised.

• When I sleep poorly one night, I know it will disturb my sleep schedule for the whole week.

• When I feel irritable, depressed or anxious during the day, it is mostly because I did not sleep well the night before.

• I feel as if insomnia is ruining my ability to enjoy life and preventing me from doing what I want.

• My sleep is getting worse all the time, and sometimes I feel as if there's not much anyone can do to help.

• I often fall asleep while watching TV, but am unable to return to sleep when I go to my bedroom.

• I get overwhelmed by my thoughts at night, and often feel that I have no control over my racing mind.

• I cannot sleep well without sleep medication.

• I have tried just about everything there is to try for insomnia, and nothing works.

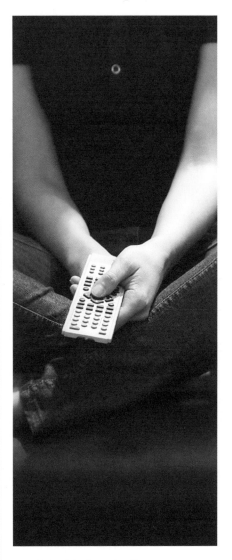

ABOVE *Late-night channel surfing is usually not as relaxing as sitting down to read a book.*

## ADDRESSING AN UNHELPFUL THOUGHT

The main point of cognitive therapy is to get rid of those thoughts that are unhelpful and potentially harming your ability to sleep better. Some of the thoughts and beliefs that you hold about sleep or insomnia may be well justified but others may be faulty and need to be corrected. For instance, you have probably gathered by now that a thought such as, 'When I have trouble getting to sleep, I should stay in bed and try harder', runs counter to CBT principles. Trying to sleep is counter-productive and simply leads to more wakefulness. When this thought occurs at 2 a.m. it may be difficult to reason against it; it needs to be countered with something like, 'That book says that I should get out of bed when I am not sleeping, and I guess I'd better stick with the programme.'

There are a variety of ways to combat these thoughts and beliefs. Practising alternatives to these thoughts during the day (either in your mind or by writing them down) will give you better access to these counter-arguments at times when you may not be thinking as clearly as you are now. The next step in the process is to come up with counter-arguments for each of the thoughts you have ticked off on the list on the previous page.

## CALCULATING THE TRUE ODDS

One approach to dealing with thoughts such as, 'If I don't get enough sleep tonight, I will mess up [fill in the blank] tomorrow', is to do a bit of arithmetic about the real probabilities of the feared event. Let's assume, for instance, that a woman we will call Mary has seriously messed up at work twice in recent years. In her sleep-deprived mind tonight, she is 94 per cent certain that she will mess up tomorrow. Mary has had insomnia for three years, and on average has about four bad nights a week. This means that she has had about 600 bad nights (4 nights x 50 weeks x 3 years), with two bad work events. This equates to a 0.33 per cent error rate. So Mary is 94 per cent certain that an event that occurs less than 1 per cent of the time will occur tomorrow. She may be right, but it is far more likely that she is worrying excessively about a low-probability event. Having done this exercise, when this thought occurs again next week, Mary can let it go and can focus on her ability to function well at work 99 per cent of the time, even with insomnia.

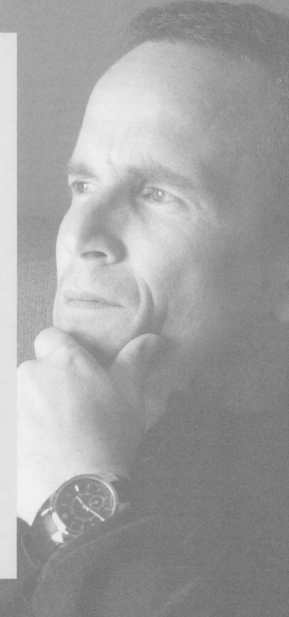

## Challenging the Thought

Some thoughts or beliefs are not so easily displaced, and a more thorough strategy is needed. One very useful approach is to run through a list of questions to ask yourself about such thoughts or beliefs:

• What evidence do I have for this thought?

• Is there any alternative way of looking at the situation?

• Is there an alternative explanation?

• How would someone else think about the situation?

• Am I setting an unrealistic standard for myself?

• Am I forgetting relevant facts or focusing too much on irrelevant facts?

• Is this an example of 'all-or-nothing' or 'black-and-white' thinking?

• If this is true, what does it mean? What would be so bad about that?

• How will things look, seem or work in a few months?

• What are the real and probable consequences of the situation?

• Am I underestimating what I can do to deal with the problem or situation?

• Am I confusing a low-probability event with one of high probability?

• Where is the logic in this thought?

• What are the advantages and disadvantages of thinking this way?

## RELAXATION TRAINING

Because insomnia often includes excessive arousal of the mind or body, introducing some form of relaxation training is a natural part of an insomnia treatment programme. As discussed in the last chapter, a number of approaches can be used to achieve relaxation. The optimal technique is largely based on individual preference and what is easiest to learn and, most importantly, which technique can be practised regularly. For those with a lot of body or muscle tension, a technique that reduces this tension will be important. For those with overactive minds, more meditative and mind-soothing techniques may be preferable. In practice, however, most relaxation techniques tend to achieve both aims quite well.

INSTRUCTIONS & IMPLEMENTATION
Start by choosing one relaxation technique and begin to practise it right away.

## A Simple Relaxation Exercise

Wearing comfortable clothes, find a quiet place to sit in a chair, with your feet on the floor, your hands in your lap, and your posture straight (though if you prefer slouching back into a recliner, go ahead).

Close your eyes and notice how you are breathing (fast, slow, or normal; deep, shallow, or in between). Without consciously changing the way you are breathing, continue to observe how you are breathing for several breaths.

Next, when you inhale, count by saying 'in one' and when you exhale, say 'out one'. Continue to count your breaths: in two, out two; in three, out three. See if you can get to ten. Most likely you will lose track somewhere. When this happens, start again at one. Do not concern yourself when your mind wanders. Simply return to counting until your mind wanders off again.

Repeat a few times until you can't quite stand it, then count for a few breaths more. Notice how you are breathing now. Slowly open your eyes. Notice how your body feels. Notice how your mind feels. Repeat daily for the next 20 years.

## Tips for Relaxation Exercises

• Choose a time and place where you will not be disturbed by family, pets, phones and so on.

This time should not be anywhere close to your bedtime while you are learning the routine.

• Start slowly and gradually. Five minutes is a reasonable length of time for your initial efforts.

• Have limited expectations. Don't expect to attain enlightenment during your first meditation, or to put your leg behind your head during your first yoga exercise. In fact, expect not to feel relaxed at all, to make what you think are mistakes and to be unsure as to how to do it 'right'.

• Practise every day.

• Gradually increase your time to 20 minutes per day (don't fret if you don't get there).

• Understand that the benefits of relaxation are cumulative; over time you will begin to notice these benefits.

• Remember the goal is not necessarily to guarantee good sleep every night. Instead, the aim of relaxation practice is to decrease your arousal levels, which will contribute to better sleep over time.

The hard work of preparing for your journey to improved sleep is nearly complete. In this final chapter, you will pull together all the homework you have been doing, as well as the evaluations and assessments I have asked you to complete, into one comprehensive tool. At your fingertips you will have as thorough a picture of your sleep problems as can be achieved. With this profile in hand, you will finalize your treatment programme and develop specific goals and a plan of action to attain them. As you begin and continue your personal sleep programme, you will record progress and address the minor problems that are bound to arise. We will also discuss how to maintain your well-earned sleep.

# CHAPTER 8
# PERSONAL SLEEP PROGRAMME

# WHAT MY SLEEP CHECKLIST & SLEEP LOG TELL ME

In previous chapters you will have completed (or at least read through) a number of descriptions, checklists and questionnaires and should have begun to keep a sleep log. It is now time to condense all this work into a comprehensive sleep checklist that captures the nature of your sleep, your sleep patterns, the initial and current causes of your insomnia and the factors that may be contributing to its chronicity.

## COMPILING THE SLEEP CHECKLIST

Opposite is a condensed version of the checklist to give you a sense of how to proceed. Using this as a draft or using the full version, first list any ongoing medical conditions or medications that you are taking, and remember to check with your doctor to make certain that these are being optimally managed and that the programme you are developing will not interfere with these conditions or medications. Also, refer back to Chapter 2 to verify that you do not have another sleep disorder, which should be addressed before commencing your programme. Use Chapter 3 to identify your type, and possible subtypes, of insomnia.

Draw heavily from Chapter 5, gleaning all the information from your sleep history and the nature of your insomnia. Also list all your current health and lifestyle factors on the sleep checklist. Describe your weekly and nightly sleep routines. Identify the sleep-hygiene factors, environmental bedroom factors, body and mind factors and specific thoughts and beliefs (from Chapter 7) that may be contributing to making your bedroom environment toxic for sleep.

## INTERPRETING SLEEP LOGS

From your two-week graphic sleep logs (see pages 112–113), you should create a list of the patterns of sleep that you can identify, then use this list to refine the description of your sleep and insomnia. If you have not yet completed a full week of the numerical sleep log, it is imperative that you do so. Once you have your weekly averages, enter them on the checklist. With this data you can also begin to keep summary graphs of your sleep variables. You should try to record your sleep variables each week.

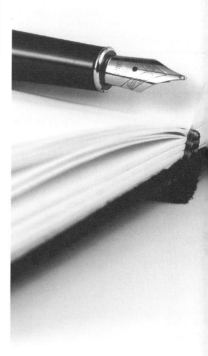

BELOW *Get into the habit of keeping accurate records, and keep your averages and checklists up to date, so that you can monitor your progress.*

### My Sleep Checklist

Existing medical conditions, current status and treatment: ...........................................

Existing medications: ..................................................

Sleep history: ............................................................

Insomnia type and subtype: .......................................

Initial and ongoing causes: ........................................

Sleep patterns: ..........................................................

Weekly and nightly routine: ......................................

Lifestyle factors: .........................................................

Sleep-hygiene factors: ...............................................

Environmental factors: ...............................................

Body and mind factors: ..............................................

Thoughts and beliefs factors: .....................................
..................................................................................

Sleep variables (weekly averages): .............................

Bedtime and rise time: ..............................................

Minutes to fall asleep: ...............................................

Number of awakenings: .............................................

Time awake during the night: ....................................

Total sleep time: ........................................................

Sleep efficiency: .........................................................

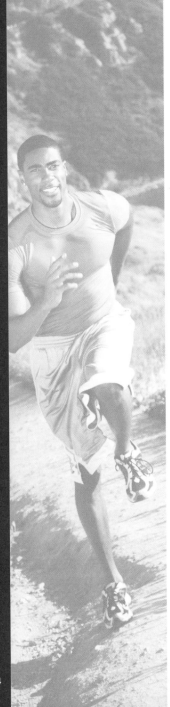

# CHECKLIST OF POTENTIAL STRATEGIES

Your sleep checklist provides a detailed view of your sleep problem, which we can now supplement with a 'Potential Strategies Checklist'. If you have already begun some of the strategies discussed in Chapter 5, you should still list them and give yourself the satisfaction of seeing progress already under way. This exercise of listing possible strategies lays the foundation for the development of your sleep programme.

### LAYING THE FOUNDATION

In the box on the opposite page is an example of what the start of a strategy list may look like. Note that it begins with a column for identifying a target problem or factor. The second column is for listing strategies that you could use to target this factor. It is very likely that some strategies will be used for more than one identified factor – this is fine. In fact, you want to make sure that you cover as many areas as possible, because insomnia can have so many contributing factors. Complete the entire list and include all possible strategies that you can find in this manual or think of on your own. Do not dismiss any strategy as too outlandish – this is a brainstorming session. Do not immediately choose a strategy.

### PERSONAL PROS & CONS OF STRATEGIES

When you have created what is probably a multiple-page document, go back to the top of the list and start writing out pros and cons for each strategy that you have written down. Again, the example on the next page indicates how this process works.

LEFT *Increasing physical activity is a useful addition to most programmes. What are the pros and cons to adding exercise to your programme?*

**Potential Strategies Checklist**

The Potential Strategies Checklist is the next to last exercise in developing a sleep programme. Complete each step of this process.

**Step 1**: Have your Detoxification Plan and your Sleep Checklist available.

**Step 2**: Start listing target factors. You can list again the problems identified in your Detoxification Plan (or not). Be sure to add sleep hygiene and lifestyle factors that you chose not to address immediately in your detoxification plan.

**Step 3**: As explained in Chapter 7, brainstorm all potential strategies to address each target factor/problem.

**Step 4**: List the pros and cons of each possible strategy for each target factor.

**Step 5**: Once the entire list is complete, weigh the pros and cons and circle those strategies that you choose to undertake.

**Step 6**: Go next to the Goals & Action Plan, which will be your treatment programme.

*Here are a couple of examples to help you get started:*

| Target Factor | Potential Strategies | Pros | Cons |
|---|---|---|---|
| 1. Spouse's snoring keeps me awake | a. Sleep in separate room | Solves problem | Not appealing |
| | b. Wear earplugs | Easy, might work | Not comfortable |
| | c. Ask your spouse to get it treated | Good for both of us | Spouse has to agree |
| | d. File for divorce | Appealing | Only joking |

| Target Factor | Potential Strategies | Pros | Cons |
|---|---|---|---|
| 2. Takes me hours to fall asleep | a. Change bedtime routine | Easy | None |
| | b. Sleep medication | Might work | Expense |
| | c. Stimulus control | Logical | Hate getting up |
| | d. Sleep restriction | Effective | Later bedtime |

*Now list yours under the following headings:*

| Target Factor | Potential Strategies | Pros | Cons |
|---|---|---|---|
| | | | |

| Target Factor | Potential Strategies | Pros | Cons |
|---|---|---|---|
| | | | |

# GOALS & PLAN OF ACTION

With your exhaustive research concluded and your strategy deliberations conducted, you are now (finally) ready to choose a course of action. In this regard, you can consider yourself a head coach finalizing a game plan, a commander deciding battle tactics or a board director launching a new company initiative. This is where you pull all the pieces together to create your own personalized sleep programme.

### PICKING A WINNING SET OF STRATEGIES

Returning to your Strategy list, take each factor one at a time and weigh up the pros and cons of each strategy you have identified. Choose one or more strategies to use for each target factor listed. Do not feel daunted if you have a particularly exhaustive list of strategies. On closer inspection you may find that many of the strategies are things that you only have to do

BELOW *Once all possible strategies are identified, it's time to pick and prioritize – but do not create undue stress by feeling that you need to start everything during the first week.*

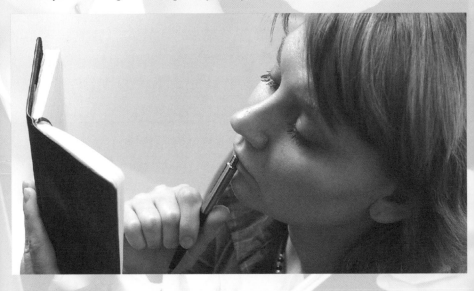

once. Some of the strategies to detoxify the sleep environment, such as turning the room temperature down at night, are quickly achieved. In addition, there is usually a sensible way to put the full programme into effect in manageable stages.

PRIORITIZING & SEQUENCING

The Detoxifying and Sleep-hygiene strategies are the best way to start (especially if you have this process underway). If you have many of these strategies listed, you can add a few new ones each week. If you have chosen sleep restriction and/or stimulus control, these are best initiated fairly early on. Stimulus control can begin right away, and sleep restriction can start as soon as you have a week's worth of sleep logs to calculate your average total sleep time for the week. The relaxation strategy you have chosen is something that can begin at any time, but the sooner it starts, the sooner the benefits of relaxation will begin to accrue.

ACTION PLAN

Create your final plan in a written version. For each target factor you have chosen to work on, list a reasonable goal, the strategy and, very importantly, the steps and time frame required to put the strategy into practice as depicted in the example below. By 'reasonable goal' I mean something that is meaningful and attainable for you. For instance, a goal of sleeping eight hours nightly, if you have not achieved this since adolescence, is probably setting the bar a little too high. Alternatively, reducing your caffeine intake from 12 cups of coffee per day to ten is probably not going to make any meaningful difference to your sleep. You get the idea. Once the plan is complete, you can readjust the timing of the strategies so that they are spaced apart in a reasonable fashion.

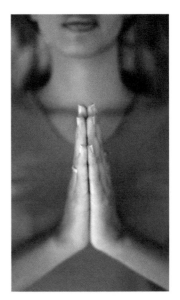

ABOVE *The sooner you begin your relaxation programme, the sooner you will reap its benefits.*

**Creating Your Action Plan**

| Target | Goal | Strategy | Steps | Time Frame |
|---|---|---|---|---|
| Excessive Time in Bed | 90 % Sleep Efficiency | Sleep Restriction | 1-Week Sleep Log | Week 1 |
| | | | Set Sleep Window | Week 2 |
| | | | Weekly Logs | Ongoing |

## KEEPING TABS & MAKING GRAPHS

As I have already indicated, keeping track of your progress is not only incredibly useful, but tends to be a strategy in and of itself. By continuing to return to your Action Plan and checking off what you have done, you will gain a sense of increased control, even before your sleep begins to improve. At the same time you will be gaining new insights into your sleep patterns. You might even notice that one or more strategies are particularly helpful. Even if you have tried them before with little success, engaging in a strategy on a consistent basis in the context of a bigger programme is often a recipe for new success.

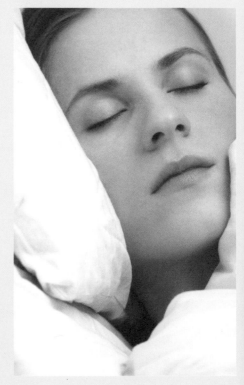

BELOW *Sleep may improve slowly in the early phases of your programme; during this time, recording your progress is a great way to help you maintain your momentum.*

### DO NOT EXPECT AN IMPROVEMENT OVERNIGHT

It is not uncommon for your total sleep time to take the longest to begin to show steady improvement, particularly when using sleep restriction, but other variables tend to improve during the first few weeks of the programme. It is also not uncommon to have some nice-looking improvements on your sleep graphs, but only modest improvements in how you feel. This is because it can take some time for the benefits of improved sleep to begin to show. It is important, therefore, to highlight even small gains that you notice in the early stages of your programme and to know that this is normally an indication that your programme is unfolding along expected lines.

## A PROBLEM-SOLVING APPROACH

The method that you used to develop your strategies and action plan can also be applied whenever you encounter a problem in the programme. For instance, you may be practising stimulus control as instructed, but find that you do not become tired. Recast the problem as 'not tired when out of bed' and come up with some strategies to address it. Perhaps you are watching television when you get out of bed and end up feeling exhausted, but not sleepy. Or perhaps you use the time out of bed to finish some home project, to surf on the Internet or to read an overly exciting piece of fiction. Seek alternatives to these and work out how to apply them. Any good plan will encounter some unforeseen problems, so the appropriate strategy is to not worry when they occur and to use the tools at your disposal to counter them.

BELOW *Approach small problems creatively. For example, if practising relaxation is difficult, try listening to music or a narrated book keeping your eyes closed.*

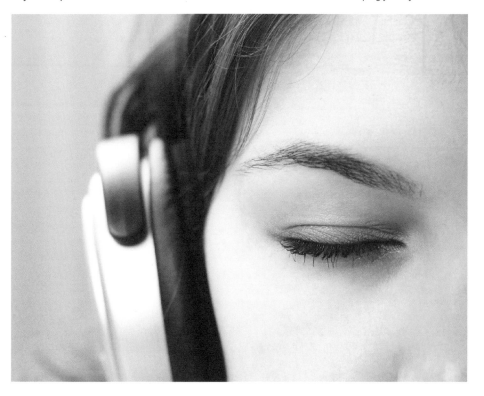

169

## MAINTENANCE & RELAPSE PREVENTION

Once you begin to see some much-desired improvements in your sleep, it may be tempting to back away from your action plan. Just like the importance of taking a full course of antibiotics, even if you begin to feel better, it is critical to continue to engage in your programme as planned. You have undertaken considerable effort to get to this point; ending your programme prematurely may put all that effort and the hard-won gains in jeopardy. So endeavour to complete the programme that you designed, and continue to implement key strategies on a long-term basis.

### ON THE VIRTUE OF PERSISTENCE

As I have now stated repeatedly, the value of consistent practice cannot be overemphasized. The brain and body love consistency. Remember that the sleep system is tightly regulated and the many sleep strategies we have covered help the sleep train to run on time. Insomnia is a persistent problem, so you must persistently engage in the strategies that combat it in order for good sleep to become a persistent state.

### MAINTAINING MOMENTUM

Quite intuitively, the best way to maintain momentum is to keep following your action plan. Completing the weekly homework review and keeping your charts updated will help you stay on track. Expect occasional setbacks to occur and meet them with continued resolve and the knowledge that you have a sound plan, and that good sleep is just another night away. At some point, usually after about two months of consistent practice (sometimes sooner and sometimes later), you will be quite pleased with your progress. At this stage you can consider whether you need to continue to fill out the daily sleep logs and tracking your progress. You will want to continue using those strategies that you have found to be most effective. Hopefully, many of these strategies will have become ingrained and it will no longer be an effort to practise them. Instead, you will find that you do not spend as much time worrying about your sleep. Sleep will take its proper place in your life.

### Preventing Occasional Poor Sleep from Becoming Persistent Insomnia

**1.** Get out of bed if you are awake for more than 10–15 minutes or when you feel annoyed, anxious, worried, frustrated and so on.

**2.** Avoid the temptation to compensate for a bad night by sleeping in, napping or going to bed early.

**3.** Keep a regular sleep schedule.

**4.** Don't allow the bed to be a place where you think or worry, or the middle of the night to be a time to solve problems.

**5.** Remember: if not tonight, then tomorrow night – you may sleep poorly tonight, but tomorrow night you're more likely to sleep well.

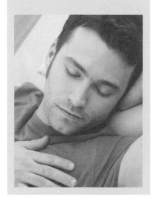

## PREVENTING A RELAPSE

Since sleep is such a sensitive system, it is quite likely that you will experience brief episodes of insomnia at various times in your life. However, do not panic when this occurs. Guard against old thought patterns that try to convince you that you are back to square one and that insomnia will return in full force. Instead, realize that this is a common occurrence in the human condition. This is not a relapse, it is just an acute episode of insomnia. Review some of the sleep strategies that were successful, and make adjustments if you are no longer using some of these tools. Remember, too, the guidelines given on the previous page.

*BELOW Once you have achieved fairly consistent good sleep, remember that the odd night of poor sleep doesn't necessarily mean a relapse into insomnia.*

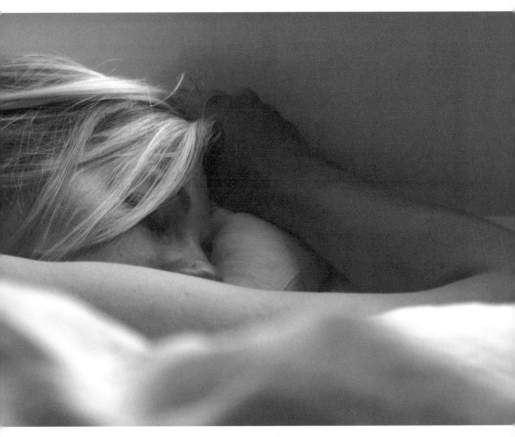

# RESOURCES

## SLEEP PRODUCTS

The online resources for sleep-related products, such as bright light boxes, devices to treat sleep apnoea, medications and alternative therapies, are too numerous to list. I encourage all readers to visit the sites hosted by the specific patient-education organizations listed below, which all have useful links to such products.

### PATIENT AND PUBLIC-EDUCATION ORGANIZATIONS

Sleep Apnoea Trust Association (SATA):
**www.sleep-apnoea-trust.org**

Managed entirely by volunteers, SATA seeks to improve the lives of sleep apnoea patients, their partners and family. The charity is dedicated to educating the public about this common disorder.

British Snoring & Sleep Apnoea Association (BSSAA):
**www.britishsnoring.co.uk**

A non-profit organization founded in 1991 that seeks to help with snoring and sleep apnoea. Its aim is to promote public awareness and help with answers to specific questions.

**www.cpap.co.uk**

Another non-profit website that provides information on new products and offers a forum for interaction with other sufferers.

International Association for the Study of Dreams:
**www.asdreams.org/index.htm**

This organization is a professional association for dream researchers, the public, and for students interested in dreams. The site is full of information.

Narcolepsy UK:
**www.narcolepsy.org.uk**

The Narcolepsy network's primary focus is to improve the lives of those with narcolepsy. Its members are people who have narcolepsy or related sleep disorders, such as idiopathic hypersomnia, plus their families and friends, and professionals involved in treatment, research, and public education regarding narcolepsy.

## THE SLEEP COUNCIL
**www.sleepcouncil.com**
A website providing general advice on the importance of a good night's sleep.

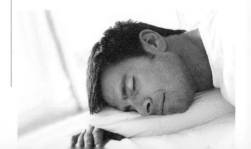

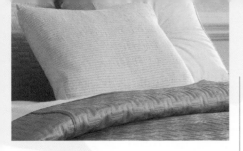

## PROFESSIONAL ORGANIZATIONS

American Academy of Sleep Medicine (AASM):
**www.aasmnet.org**

This is the membership academy for sleep professionals in the United States, although many sleep professionals from other countries are also members. It is the world's largest professional sleep organization. The site is geared primarily toward members and other health-care professionals, but also includes useful patient information.

### BRITISH SLEEP SOCIETY
**www.sleeping.org.uk**

A professional organization that aims to improve public health and sleep education. All members have an interest in sleep disorders.

### THE LONDON SLEEP CENTRE
**www.thelondonsleepcentre.com**

A professional organization that provides diagnostic and treatment services for people with sleep disorders.

**www.osauk.org/osauk**

A commercial website providing information on sleep disorders.

World Federation of Sleep Research & Sleep Medicine Societies (WSF):
**www.wfsrsms.org**

The WSF facilitates international collaborations and cooperation among professional sleep societies around the world and promotes sleep health as a worldwide public-health priority. There is some patient information on the member sites, although the sites are primarily geared toward sleep professionals. Member societies include the AASM, the CSS, the Sleep Research Society (**www.sleepresearchsociety. org**), the European Sleep and Research Society (**www.esrs.eu**), the Australian Sleep Society (**www.sleepaus.on.net**), the Asian Sleep Research Society (**www.asrsonline.org**), and the Federation of Latin American Sleep Societies (**icb.usp.br/~flass/index2.html**).

## BOOKS

*Sleep* by J. Allan Hobson (W.H. Freeman, 1995)

This wonderful book by a pioneering sleep researcher provides some fascinating reading on the science of sleep, and does so with visually pleasing photographs and artwork.

*The Sleepwatchers* by William C. Dement (Nychthemeron Press, 1996)

This is essentially a combination of an anecdotal autobiography and a wide-ranging trip through sleep and sleep disorders by one of the pioneers of sleep medicine and sleep research.

# INDEX

# ACKNOWLEDGEMENTS

**Author's acknowledgements**

To my mentor in sleep medicine, Michael Sateia, your wisdom and guidance have been profound and remain profoundly appreciated.

To my mentors in sleep research, Tom Mellman and Michael Perlis, your training and support have been invaluable and I value them greatly.

To my life mentor and partner, Catherine Faurot, your steadfast love and support promote successes on all fronts and I cherish them, and you.

To our four sons, Patrick, Galen, Conor and Taran, the lives you lead make ours a wonderful adventure.

The publishers would like to thank Dr Stephen Lund for his helpful input in the editing of this work.

The publishers would also like to thank the following people and organizations for permission to use the images in this book:

**Alamy**/Arco Images GmbH: 131cr; TH Foto: 131tr.

**Alan Osbahr:** 3.

**Corbis**/Envision: 14; Zena Holloway: 48; Nick North: 86; Simon Jarratt: 96; Eric Audras: 101; JGI: 146.

**Fotolia:** 28; Mat Hayward: 33; Kurhan: 54; Alena Yakusheva: 115; Valua Vitaly: 175, 176.

**Getty Images**/Time & Life Pic
Still Images: 62; D E Cox: 72;
Mittongtare: 118; James Dar
Scott E Barbour: 133.

**iStockphoto**/Neustockimage
60, 67, 71br, 74, 98, 99bl, 10?
147, 163; Tomm L: 6, 45br, 7?
Cole: 9c; Jacob Wackerhause
Oleg Prikhodko: 10, 13bl; Ma...
Barsse: 11, 108r; Nick Schlax: 12; Rich
Legg: 13r; Imelda Kiss: 19; Ekaterina
Monakhova: 20b; Jente Kasprowski: 23; Justin Horrocks: 25c, cover; 30; Anna Bryukhanova: 33; Nathan Gleave: 40; Michael DeLeon: 44; 47; Webphotographer: 51; 53; Roberto Caucino: 57; Anna Lubovedskaya: 58; June Cairns: 59; 62; 71t; 75; 76; Juan Monino: 78tr; Andrew Rich: 82; 84; Roberta Casaliggi: 85; 89; Alexander Shalamov: 91; Leon Tura: 94; R C Young: 96tr; jean Frooms: 99br; Amanda Rohde: 104; Catherine Yeulet: 108l; Noel Powell: 109; VikaValter: 110, 168tr; Stephan Popov: 112; Daniel Bendjy: 118b; Kristian Sekulic: 120; 121; Daniella Zalcman: 125c; Darren Baker: 125tr; Amanda Rohde: 127br, 137tr; Denise Torres: 127l; 130; 131; Rafal Zdeb: 132; Jeff Edney: 133tr; Marcus Clackson: 134br; PlainView: 135; Andrew Johnson: 137br; Skip ODonnell: 138b; Agnes Csondor: 138cr; EauClaire Media: 140; Sharon Dominick: 141br; 143; 148; Hanna Maria H: 149; Lumenphoto: 153b; FreezeFrameStudio: 153t; David

...in Sleep (1996), 19 (8), P ??9,
95, 97 (data taken from a Gallup poll for the National Sleep Foundation, 2002), 100 (adapted from Perlis, M.L., Giles, D.E., Buysse, D.J., Tu, X., Kupfer, D.J., (1997) 'Self-reported sleep disturbance as a prodromal symptom in recurrent depression'. J Affective Disorders (42, 2,3): 209–212), 102, 150 (Adapted from Spielman, A., Caruso, L., and Glovinsky, P. (1987), 'A behavioral perspective on insomnia treatment'. Psychiatr. Clin. North Am. 10 (4): 541–553), 151 (Adapted from Perlis, M., Smith, M., and Pigeon, W. (2005) 'Etiological perspectives of insomnia' in Kryger M., Roth T., and Dement, W. (eds) Principles and Practice of Sleep Medicine, 4th edn. Philadelphia: WB Saunders.)

**NASA:** 73.

**Photos.com:** 22, 29, 32, 37, 38, 39, 45, 47, 53, 64, 66, 75, 87, 121, 122, 142, 150, 151, 155, 166, 169.

**Richard Peters:** 21, 49, 70.

**Science Photo Library**/National Library of Medicine: 34t.